Visit our website

to find out about other books from W.B. Saunders
and our sister companies in Harcourt Health Sciences

Register free at
www.harcourt-international.com

D0202065

and you will get

- **the latest information on new books, journals and electronic products in your chosen subject areas**

- **the choice of e-mail or post alerts or both, when there are any new books in your chosen areas**

- **news of special offers and promotions**

- **information about products from all Harcourt Health Sciences companies including W. B. Saunders, Churchill Livingstone, and Mosby**

You will also find an easily searchable catalogue, online ordering, information on our extensive list of journals...and much more!

Visit the Harcourt Health Sciences website today!

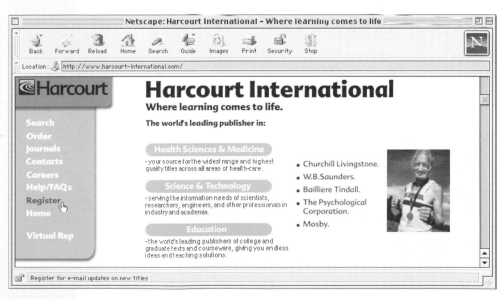

Harcourt
Health Sciences

Pain Management in Animals

Commissioning Editor: Deborah Russell
Project Editor: Rolla Couchman
Production Manager: Helen Sofio
Design Manager: Jayne Jones

Pain Management in Animals

Edited by

Paul A. Flecknell MA VetMB PhD
DLAS DiplECVA MRCVS

Professor of Laboratory Animal Science and Director
Comparative Biology Centre
The Medical School
University of Newcastle-upon-Tyne
Newcastle-upon-Tyne, United Kingdom

Avril Waterman-Pearson BVSc PhD
FRCVS DVA DiplECVA

Professor of Veterinary Anaesthesia and Head of Department
Department of Clinical Veterinary Science
University of Bristol
Bristol, United Kingdom

 W. B. SAUNDERS

London • Edinburgh • New York • Philadelphia • St Louis • Sidney • Toronto 2000

WB SAUNDERS
An imprint of Harcourt Publishers Limited

First published 2000

ISBN 0 7020 1767 1

British Library Cataloguing in Publication Data
A catalogue record for this book is available from the British Library

Library of Congress Cataloging in Publication Data
A catalogue record for this book is available from the Library of Congress

Note
Medical knowledge is constantly changing. As new information becomes available, changes in treatment, procedures, equipment and the use of drugs become necessary. The editors and contributors and the publishers have taken care to ensure that the information given in this text is accurate and up to date. However, readers are strongly advised to confirm that the information, especially with regard to drug usage, complies with the latest legislation and standards of practice.

The
publisher's
policy is to use
**paper manufactured
from sustainable forests**

Printed by Bell & Bain Ltd., Glasgow
Typeset by Kolam, India

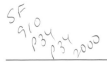

Preface

Although all veterinary surgeons share a common concern for the welfare of animals under their care, the prevention and alleviation of pain has not always been implemented effectively. Misconceptions about the nature and significance of pain, difficulties in recognising its severity and uncertainty as to the most appropriate therapy have all hampered progress in this area. This book sets out to address some of these obstacles by bringing together current thinking concerning the recognition and management of pain. In order to manage pain effectively, some knowledge of the underlying physiological processes and the pharmacology of analgesics are essential, so concise summaries of these areas are provided. The contributors have tried to provide information on as wide a range of species as possible, and to encompass a variety of different clinical scenarios, but have been hampered by the fundamental lack of scientific data in many of these areas. Despite these limitations, which we hope will be remedied by future research, this book aims to provide practical information that will be of value to all those concerned with pain management in animals. The contributors have tried to dispel some of the myths surrounding analgesic use – for example that opioids cannot be given to cats and to provide soundly based recommendations for pain therapy.

We have been fortunate in obtaining contributions from colleagues with a wide breadth of clinical experience, obtained both in university and referral centres, and general veterinary practice. Inevitably, opinions differed in some areas, notably in the most appropriate dose rates of analgesics. These have been resolved by providing a broad dose range for most drugs in the various tables, and encouraging clinicians to assess the effects of these agents and administer additional doses as required. Since this is a rapidly developing field, we would advise that analgesic dose rates are always compared with current recommendations from their manufacturers, when veterinary products are available.

We hope that this book will provide a convenient and practically useful summary of current concepts of pain management in animals. We hope it will encourage wider and more effective use of analgesics in animals, and particularly to their use not simply for post-surgical or post-traumatic pain control, but also for other conditions in which pain may be experienced.

We would like to thank our colleagues for their support and encouragement, the secretarial staff at Newcastle for their help in preparing the manuscript and the editorial staff at Harcourt Publishers for their patience during the production of this book.

Paul Flecknell
Avril Waterman-Pearson
2000

Contents

Contributors

Malcolm J. Brearley MA VetMB
  MSc(ClinOnc) FRCVS
Davies White Veterinary Specialists
Higham Gobion, Hertfordshire,
United Kingdom

Jacqueline C. Brearley MA VetMB
  PhD DVA DiplECVA MRCVS
Animal Health Trust
Newmarket, Suffolk, United
  Kingdom

Paul Chambers BVSc PhD DVA
  MRCVS
Senior Lecturer in Clinical
Pharmacology
Institute of Veterinary, Animal and
  Biomedical Sciences
Massey University
Palmerston North, New Zealand

Petro Dobromylskyj BSc BVetMed
  DVA DiplECVA MRCVS
Broadland House Veterinary
  Surgery
Stalham, Norfolk, United Kingdom

Paul Flecknell MA VetMB PhD
  DLAS DiplECVA MRCVS
Professor of Laboratory Animal
Science and Director
Comparative Biology Centre
The Medical School
University of Newcastle-upon-Tyne
Newcastle-upon-Tyne, United
  Kingdom

B. Duncan X. Lascelles BSc
  BVSc(Hons) PhD MRCVS
  CertVA DSAS(ST) DiplECVS
Lecturer in Small Animal Surgery
Department of Clinical Veterinary
  Science
Bristol University
Bristol, United Kingdom

Alexander Livingston BSc BVetMed
  PhD FRCVS
Professor of Pharmacology
Dean, Western College of Veterinary
  Medicine
University of Saskatchewan
Saskatoon, Saskatchewan, Canada

Andrea M. Nolan MVB MRCVS
  DVA PhD DiplECVA DipEVCPT
Professor of Veterinary
  Pharmacology
Faculty of Veterinary Medicine
University of Glasgow
Glasgow, United Kingdom

Peter J. Pascoe BVSc DVA DipACVA
  DiplECVA MRCVS
Professor of Anesthesiology
Department of Surgical and
  Radiological Sciences
School of Veterinary Medicine
University of California
Davis, California, USA

Polly M. Taylor MAVet MB PhD
  DVA DiplECVA MRCVS
University Lecturer in Anaesthesia
Department of Clinical Veterinary
  Medicine
University of Cambridge
Cambridge, United Kingdom

Avril Waterman-Pearson BVSc PhD
  FRCVS DVA DiplECVA
Professor of Veterinary Anaesthesia
  and Head of Department
Department of Clinical Veterinary
  Science
University of Bristol
Bristol, United Kingdom

ANIMAL PAIN – AN INTRODUCTION

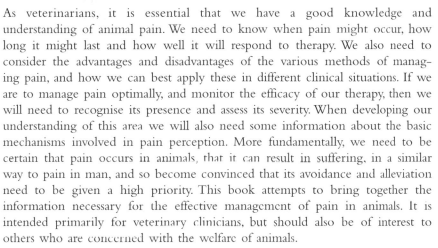

P. A. Flecknell

As veterinarians, it is essential that we have a good knowledge and understanding of animal pain. We need to know when pain might occur, how long it might last and how well it will respond to therapy. We also need to consider the advantages and disadvantages of the various methods of managing pain, and how we can best apply these in different clinical situations. If we are to manage pain optimally, and monitor the efficacy of our therapy, then we will need to recognise its presence and assess its severity. When developing our understanding of this area we will also need some information about the basic mechanisms involved in pain perception. More fundamentally, we need to be certain that pain occurs in animals, that it can result in suffering, in a similar way to pain in man, and so become convinced that its avoidance and alleviation need to be given a high priority. This book attempts to bring together the information necessary for the effective management of pain in animals. It is intended primarily for veterinary clinicians, but should also be of interest to others who are concerned with the welfare of animals.

It is important to make clear at the outset that our knowledge of animal pain, and its assessment and alleviation, is still very limited. For many years, clinicians lacked information on analgesic agents and their use in animals, and our attempts at pain assessment were rudimentary. In recent years there has been a rapid increase in information, but much of it has yet to be applied to clinical practice. Despite the availability of analgesic agents, our use of them remains low in comparison to their use in man. The possible reasons for this are discussed in this introductory chapter, together with a consideration of some of the more fundamental issues concerning the nature of pain perception in animals. This is followed by two chapters discussing the physiology of pain and nociception, and the pharmacology of analgesic agents. The information in this section is developed and placed in a clinical context in the succeeding chapters, which deal with recognition and assessment of pain, pain management, management of particular clinical problems, and the difficult area of chronic pain management. Although some sections of the text can be used as a 'recipe book' for pain management, we would encourage clinicians to read all of the chapters, so that they can make the most effective use of the techniques which are described.

Animal pain and analgesic use

Most veterinary surgeons would have no hesitation in stating that animals experience pain. On reflection, they might add that the experience might not be exactly the same as the pain they might experience themselves, but nevertheless would have no doubt that was 'pain'. This assertion is supported by the results of several recent questionnaires, which established that the majority of respondents considered animals to experience pain in a range of circumstances, for example following surgery (Dohoo & Dohoo 1996 a and b, Capner et al 1999, Lascelles et al 2000). But if veterinary clinicians believe animals experience pain, why are analgesics used so infrequently in animals, compared to best practice in human patients? Despite the increased availability of analgesic agents for use in animals, only 50% of dogs and cats receive analgesics after ovariohysterectomy, and only 23% of small mammals after major surgery (Capner et al 1999, Lascelles et al 2000). Although analgesic and antiinflammatory drugs are widely used to treat arthritis and other musculoskeletal conditions in horses and companion animals, analgesics are rarely used in other medical conditions which are likely to cause pain, for example neoplasia, mastitis and otitis externa. It seems appropriate, then, to examine some of the assumptions we make about animal pain, and to assess whether these influence our clinical decisions.

Do animals experience pain?

Although most clinicians accept that animals experience pain, it is important that we establish a basis for this assumption. There can be no doubt that the ability to detect damaging or potentially damaging stimuli, for example excess heat or mechanical pressure, is present in many animal species. Possession of this detection system does not, in itself, mean that animals experience pain. Pain in man is recognised as having both a sensory and an emotional component. Without interpretation by the brain of the sensory information arriving from peripheral nerves, the characteristic unpleasant and distressing nature of pain is not appreciated (see chapter 2).

The initial processing of information arising in the peripheral detection system, which relates to potentially damaging stimuli, is termed 'nociception'. The interpretation of this information centrally results in the experience of pain. Animals and humans both possess nociceptors, and these receptors, and the types of nerve fibres that connect them to the central nervous system, are virtually identical in all animals. The processing of this information in the spinal cord and lower parts of the brain is also very similar, and potential differences primarily arise when the information reaches the cerebral cortex. Whether animals possess the same, or a similar, capacity as man to experience emotions such as pain has been extensively debated for centuries. The main reason for the continued debate is that it is impossible to investigate such emotional states directly – we can only draw inferences from other, indirect, measures, such as investigation of behavioural responses. Some philosophers have firmly asserted that animals cannot experience pain – the most often quoted is Descartes, who stated 'The greatest of all the prejudices we have retained from our infancy is that of believing that the beasts think' (*quoted in* Haldane & Ross 1989). Descartes asserted that since animals had no capacity for reasoning, they could have no perception of pain, and that their reactions to stimuli that would cause pain in man were simply the responses of automatons. Although there have been a number of different responses to Descartes' ideas, that of Jeremy Bentham, the 18th century utilitarian philosopher, is most frequently cited: 'The question is not can they reason? Nor can the talk? But can they suffer?' (*quoted in* Bowring 1962). Most clinicians would accept Bentham's view that animals *can* suffer, and reject the idea that their responses were simply reflexes, with no conscious perception.

Scientific support for this belief would often consist simply of drawing parallels in animal and human neuroanatomy, and making the suggestion that animals 'are given the benefit of the doubt'. When comparing the central nervous system structures believed to be associated with pain perception, or at least with the unpleasant aspect of pain, it is likely that the prefrontal cortex has an important role. In man, prefrontal lobotomy was used as a treatment for some psychiatric disorders. Patients who had undergone this procedure still responded to painful stimuli by reflex movements, but expressed no concern about their pain – it was no longer considered unpleasant. Most animal species have relatively small areas of prefrontal cortex, and this has led to the suggestion that pain in animals is comparable to that experienced by lobotomised humans (Melzack & Dennis 1980, Bermond 1997). This assumes that absolute size of the prefrontal cortex will determine the capacity for pain perception, but it may be that other areas of the brain carry out a similar role in non-human species (Divac et al 1993). What is clear, however, is that animals do not behave in simple, reflex ways, in circumstances that would cause pain in man.

Animals and their response to pain

Aside from immediate avoidance or defence reactions, such as struggling or biting when an injured limb is handled, animals show a range of more subtle behavioural responses to pain. Animals can be trained to perform complex tasks to avoid brief painful stimuli, and other studies have shown that animals can choose to self-administer analgesics when they develop chronic painful conditions (Colpaert 1987, Danbury et al in press). The response to an analgesic has often been used to determine whether a behaviour was pain related, and although it can become a circular argument (animal pain behaviour is behaviour modified by analgesic drugs, which are drugs that alleviate pain), it provides some useful information when developing pain assessment schemes for animals. The development of assessment schemes is of central importance to our understanding and appreciation of animal pain. If we cannot assess pain, we cannot manage it effectively, and it is likely that a failure to appreciate the severity of pain in individual animals is the single most important factor in the apparent underuse of analgesics discussed earlier.

Most clinicians expect to be able to recognise pain in animals, and we develop clear ideas concerning responses to acute pain. Unfortunately, we retain a level of anthropomorphism which leads us to expect animals in pain to behave in the same way as humans in pain. Animals in pain might be expected to behave in different ways depending upon the site, severity and type of pain, but we should also expect them to behave in a species-specific way. Some species, especially those which may expect support from others, may show very obvious pain-related behaviour. In other species, expressing such overt behaviour would simply alert predators that they were less fit and hence easy prey. If overt pain-related behaviour is expressed, then the animal may mask this behaviour when it is aware it is being observed. Animals may also change their responses when in a familiar, secure environment, and express less pain-related behaviour when in an unfamiliar environment, such as a veterinary surgeon's consulting room! It is important, then, that we examine our preconceptions about pain behaviour critically and try to establish which clinical signs indicate the presence of pain in animals. These clinical signs are of course likely to vary in different species and with different clinical conditions.

It is important not simply to assume that conditions that are painful in man will be painful in animals, since the choice of analgesic should be influenced by the degree of pain that is actually present. If inappropriate use is made of a potent analgesic, then the undesirable side-effects of the agent may outweigh any potential beneficial pain-alleviating effects. In order to determine the degree of pain that is present, and so choose an appropriate analgesic regimen, some form of assessment is required. Without a scheme of assessment, it is necessary to assume that the degree of pain present will be identical in humans and animals in similar circumstances. A consideration of the differences in anatomy, posture and behaviour between animals and man illustrates that this assumption is unlikely to be correct. Furthermore, in order to provide effective pain relief for as long as required, if no assessment scheme is used then it is necessary to assume that the duration of pain, for example following a particular surgical procedure, will be identical in animals and man. It will also be necessary to assume that the rate of decrease in the severity of the pain is also the same. Even if these assumptions were to be true, it would also be necessary to assume that all animals will experience the same level of pain. This is patently illogical – in man, it is well established that different individuals have different analgesic requirements after apparently identical surgical procedures (Alexander & Hill 1987). In man, the dose of analgesic administered, and the frequency and duration of treatment, is adjusted by assessing pain in each individual patient. In animals, it seems reasonable to assume that effective pain relief can be achieved only by making a similar assessment. Selection of an arbitrary initial dose of analgesic is unlikely to prove uniformly effective. The response to a particular dose of an analgesic has been shown to vary considerably between animals of different strains, ages and sexes (Frommel & Joye 1964, Katz 1980, Moskowitz et al 1985). So selection of a particular dose regimen can result in over-dosage of some animals, and provision of inadequate analgesia for others. It is therefore of fundamental importance that accurate methods of assessment of pain and distress are developed, so that analgesic treatment can be tailored to suit the needs of each individual patient.

Although our ability to recognise pain in animals remains poor, adopting a critical approach has enabled pain scoring systems in dogs, cats, horses, sheep, calves and small rodents to be developed (see chapter 4). As further studies progress, it should be possible to devise systems of assessment that can be introduced successfully into veterinary practice. One important point to note is that many of these schemes are attempting to differentiate small gradations in the animals' sensation of pain. Recognising obvious clinical signs of marked pain in species such as the dog and cat is not difficult, and should result in the use of appropriate analgesic therapy.

When could pain occur?

It does not seem unreasonable to assume that since the peripheral mechanisms for detection of potentially painful stimuli are similar in animals and man, and the mechanisms for processing these signals are remarkably similar, then the circumstances that could give rise to pain will also be similar. Clearly, we must also give careful consideration to differences in anatomy, and differences in the natural environment of particular species, but broad similarities are likely to exist. If this is so, then it should influence our clinical decision-making. At present, analgesics are widely used to control pain in two groups of animals – those that have undergone surgery or have suffered traumatic injuries, and those with acute or chronic arthritis. Large groups of patients with conditions that could be associated with pain rarely receive analgesic therapy to complement the treatment of the primary condition. Any condition with a marked inflammatory component, for example an abscess following a bite, impacted or infected anal glands, otitis externa, conjunctivitis, cystitis and mastitis probably causes pain, as can conditions resulting in tissue distension or damage, for example neoplasia. In man, these or similar conditions often cause significant pain. Much of our information concerning the response of veterinary patients to analgesics in these circumstances is anecdotal, but it seems illogical to exclude them from pain management schemes. It is also clear that since many of these conditions have a marked inflammatory component, NSAIDs may well be the most appropriate analgesic therapy (see chapters 5, 6 and 7).

It has been argued that pain alleviation is not always desirable. We know that pain evolved to have a protective function, and that the presence of pain prevents or discourages use of damaged tissues, and this helps prevent further damage. This is correct, but in circumstances in which we are taking responsibility for the animal, and repairing surgical wounds appropriately, then removing the protective role of pain almost never has detrimental effects. In circumstances when specific concerns are raised, for example after major orthopaedic surgery, then additional measures such as application of supportive bandages and splints, or confinement of the animal so that it rests the injured area can be used in conjunction with administration of analgesics. It is worth noting that similar arguments can arise when treating young children who, like animals, cannot be instructed to remain still and rest after administration of pain-relieving drugs, but paediatricians do not normally withhold analgesics on these grounds, and aim to provide effective pain relief to infants as well as to adults. In any event, such arguments hinge on the idea that analgesics are so effective they remove all pain sensation – this is rarely the case, and excessive exertion of an injured body part will still provoke some of pain's warning function. In almost all circumstances, abolishing the detrimental effects of pain almost always outweighs any possible disadvantage of removing pain's protective function. Aside from being unpleasant and potentially distressing, pain can slow recovery from surgery, can reduce food and water consumption, interfere with normal respiration (for example after thoracotomy), and reduce a whole range of 'self-maintenance' behaviours. The immobility caused by pain can lead to muscle spasm, can cause atrophy of areas, and can slow healing. Prolonged immobility can also cause pressure sores, urine scalding, faeces soiling and can greatly complicate patient management. Pain can also prolong the catabolic response to trauma or surgery, and chronic pain can lead to further endocrine and metabolic changes which are generally detrimental to the animal.

There are other reasons for our frequent failure to alleviate animal pain. A lack of information as to appropriate doses of analgesics and a lack of guidance as to the choice of analgesic may lead to all analgesic therapy being withheld. It is hoped that this problem is addressed in chapters 5–7. One common reason for withholding analgesics is concern about their undesirable side-effects, particularly since many misconceptions, such as the view that morphine cannot be given to cats, are still widely held by veterinarians. Fortunately, with the growing concern amongst veterinary surgeons for the need to control animal pain, more information concerning the safe and appropriate use of analgesics is becoming available, and this is summarised in chapters 3–7. In most circumstances, the undesirable side-effects of analgesics are of little or no clinical significance. When side-effects could be a problem, then they can almost always be avoided or successfully managed by understanding the underlying reasons for their occurrence (see chapter 3).

Finally, there are a number of practical problems concerning analgesic use that can restrict their administration. In many countries, the use of the majority of opioids is controlled by legislation (the Misuse of Drugs Act 1971, in the UK). Complying with this legislation often requires careful record keeping of the purchase, storage and dispensing of opioids and may restrict the persons who are able to dispense and administer these substances. In some countries the degree of record keeping required can act as a strong disincentive. Legislative control, together with genuine safety concerns, also limit the dispensing of this class of analgesics for out-patient use. This is not an absolute contraindication, and each case should be considered separately, although clearly clinicians must observe local regulations. An additional concern is that since these are drugs of abuse, their presence in a veterinary practice may increase the likelihood of theft. It is important to place this in context, and remember that other agents such as ketamine, barbiturates and benzodiazepines are also frequently kept on veterinary premises.

References

Alexander, J.I. and Hill, R.G. (1987) *Postoperative Pain Control*. Blackwell Scientific Publications, Oxford.

Bermond, B. (1997) The myth of animal suffering. In: Dol, M. et al (eds) *Animal Consciousness and Animal Ethics*. Van Gorcum Publications, Assen, The Netherlands, pp 125–143.

Bowring, J. (ed) (1962) *The Works of Jeremy Bentham*. Russell and Russell, New York, vol. 1, pp 142–143.

Capner, C.A., Lascelles, B.D.X. and Waterman-Pearson, A.E. (1999) Current British veterinary attitudes to perioperative analgesia for dogs *Veterinary Record* **145**: 95–99.

Colpaert, F. (1987) Evidence that adjuvant arthritis in the rat is associated with chronic pain. *Pain* **28**: 201–222.

Danbury, T.C., Weeks, C., Kestin, S.C. and Waterman-Pearson, A.E. (2000) Self-selection of the analgesic drug carprofen by lame broiler chickens. *Veterinary Record* (in press).

Divac, I., Mogensen, J., Petrovic Minic, B., Zilles, K., and Regidor, J., (1993) Cortical projections of the thalamic mediodorsal nucleus in the rat. Definition of the prefrontal cortex. *Acta Neurobiologiae Experimentalis* **53**: 425–429.

Dohoo, S.E. and Dohoo, I.R. (1996a) Post-operative use of analgesics in dogs and cats by Canadian veterinarians. *Canadian Veterinary Journal* **37**: 546–551.

Dohoo, S.E. and Dohoo, I.R. (1996b) Factors influencing the postoperative use of analgesics in dogs and cats by Canadian veterinarians. *Canadian Veterinary Journal* **37**: 552–556.

Frommel, E. and Joye, E. (1964) On the analgesic power of morphine in relation to age and sex of guinea-pigs. *Medicina Experimentalis* **11**: 43–46.

Haldane, E.S. and Ross, G.R.T. (trs) (1989) Selections from discourse on method, part 5. In: *Philosophic Works of Descartes*. Cambridge University Press, London, vol. 1, pp 115–118.

Katz, R.J. (1980) The albino locus produces abnormal responses to opiates in the mouse. *European Journal of Pharmacology*, **68**: 229–232.

Lascelles, B.D.X., Capner, C.A. and Waterman-Pearson, A.E. (2000) Current British veterinary attitudes to perioperative analgesia for dogs and small mammals. *Veterinary Record* (in press).

Melzack, R. and Dennis, S.G. (1980) Phylogenetic evolution of pain-expression in animals. In: Kosterlitz, H.W. and Terenius, L.Y. (eds) *Pain and Society*, Verlag Chemie, Weinheim, Germany, pp 13–26.

Moskowitz, A.S., Terman, G.W., Carter, K.R., Morgan, M.J. and Liebeskind, J.C. (1985) Analgesic, locomotor and lethal effects of morphine in the mouse: strain comparisons. *Brain Research* **361**: 46–51.

THE PHYSIOLOGY OF PAIN

2

A. Livingston, P. Chambers

Introduction

Much of the knowledge of the physiological processes of pain perception has, for obvious ethical and welfare reasons, come from studies in anaesthetised animals. However, when you think about it, the philosophical question of whether animals can feel 'pain' and the significance of studies in anaesthetised animals, which by definition are unable to feel pain, must make us wonder about the relevance of some of the findings. These concepts, as discussed in chapter 1, have dogged the understanding of the processes involved for many years. Another factor which has confused the search for the mechanisms involved was the concept that 'pain' was a single entity and that its detection and processing was a simple 'hard-wired' system, not unlike a complicated electrical circuit (Fig. 2.1).

The concept of the reflex arc, whereby the noxious stimulus resulted in an involuntary withdrawal of the body part without the involvement of higher centres, did not help understanding of pain perception in animals, since animal pain response could be dismissed as a simple spinal reflex which did not necessarily result in any cerebral perception of pain. In man, the 'pain experience' can be separated into three components:

- transmission of the signal provoked by the noxious stimulus to the brain (nociception);
- perception of an unpleasant experience;
- the behavioural (or cognitive) response to pain.

The fundamental problem facing those wishing to study pain in animals is that pain cannot be measured – it can only be inferred. Since pain is a conceptual sense and presumably is perceived only at the highest brain centres as a result of inputs from elsewhere in the body, scientists have developed the concept of 'nociception.' Nociception refers to the sensory processes which result, in man, in the perception of pain following a noxious, or damaging, stimulus. Thus we use the term to describe the changes we see in non-verbal animals which are likely to have 'pain-like' consequences. Nociception, i.e. electrical or chemical activity in sensory neurones and receptors, can be measured, but this is not pain; it may be related, it may even be proportional, but in animals we cannot tell. Similarly, we can look at behavioural activity in animals, and like electrical activity, it can be measured and quantified. It too may be related or even

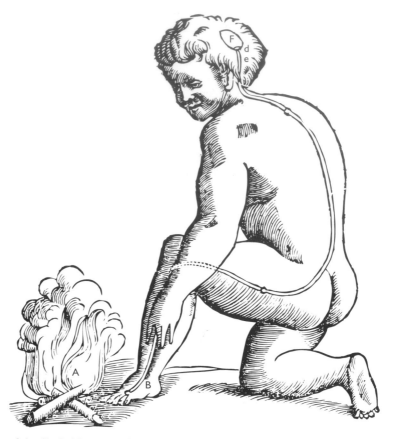

Figure 2.1. Early ideas on pain transmission. Descartes, in his *Traité de l'homme* (1664), considered that pain was transmitted by a string from the site of the stimulus to the seat of consciousness in the pineal gland. Apart from replacing the string with an electric wire, the theory did not change much until recently!

proportional, but in the same way we can only assume; we cannot tell for certain if what we are seeing and measuring is the same thing as pain. The emotional perception of something as 'unpleasant' cannot be quantified even in man and its existence in animals is denied by many.

Knowledge of the anatomical and physiological processes in the nervous system associated with pain perception in animals is further confused by examination of the situation in humans. The fact that a significant number of human patients who describe pain as a primary symptom will show no anatomical, physiological or pathological defect which could explain the pain perceived should cause those working with animals some considerable concern. Much of modern medical thinking is based on the assumption that pain is caused by a 'defect' in the neuronal or receptive system and that correction of that 'defect' will stop the pain. However, we also know that there is often no detectable 'defect' – so how do we correct it?

If this situation exists in humans, who can clearly describe the nature, location and intensity of their pain, we obviously have a very difficult situation when assessing pain in animals. However, recent advances in knowledge of the processes associated with pain allow the development of rational strategies to control pain.

Perhaps one of the most useful methods of understanding pain in all its numerous manifestations is to consider the simple separation of pain types into physiological and pathological pains (Woolf & Chong 1993). A physiological pain can be described as a means of detecting a noxious input where the perception of pain is proportional to the intensity of the noxious stimulus. This form of pain can be regarded as a defensive mechanism designed to limit the damage to the body by a noxious stimulus and as such can serve a useful purpose; it could equally well be described as 'protective' pain.

The pathological type of pain can be described as a perception that is greater than the apparent noxious stimulus. This can take several forms: for instance where the peripheral stimulus has resulted in inflammatory changes, the perception of pain can be increased, e.g. pressure on an area of traumatised skin; or chronic ongoing pain can lead to a centrally sensitised state, with an increased sensitivity to pain from other regions; or pathological pain may even take the form of neurogenic pain, where there are no lesions to provide a noxious stimulus, but the perception of pain is still there, e.g. in phantom limb pain. Each sort of pain is more likely to be treated effectively when the underlying mechanisms associated with the pain are understood.

Nociceptive mechanisms

The response to a noxious stimulus involves a number of processes. The stimulus is detected at the periphery and passed along the afferent sensory nerve fibres to the spinal cord. Some processing occurs here; then the signal is passed on to the brain. In many cases, the brain will try to suppress the signal by a descending inhibition on the spinal cord. This probably evolved to allow the animal to get away from the noxious stimulus and out of danger. Meanwhile, if the noxious stimulus was intense enough, or if it caused any tissue damage, an inflammatory reaction will have been set up. This sensitises the peripheral nerve fibres and increases the signal arriving at the cord; after a while, modulation of the signal at the cord switches from suppression to amplification. This has an evolutionary advantage by forcing the animal to rest, which encourages healing. Eventually (in most cases) sensation returns to normal. This extensive processing of the 'pain' signal allows plenty of opportunities for intervention with analgesic drugs.

Afferent pathways

The sensory nerves associated with transmission of (noxious) information which may be perceived as pain are of two distinct anatomical types: the small myelinated A (δ) fibres, usually associated with sharp mechanical type stimuli; and the unmyelinated C fibres, associated with dull, burning or longer lasting pain. The size and degree of myelination of these fibres will influence the ease of access of local analgesics to these nerves, producing some degree of gradation of effect (see chapter 5).

Under 'normal' physiological conditions a mechanical, thermal or chemical stimulus will open various ion channels to trigger the nerve ending to send afferent action potentials along the sensory A or C fibre. These action potentials are propagated by the opening of sodium channels and can be either in a continuous or burst form depending on the location or type of nerve ending, and an increased noxious stimulus will give an increase in the firing rate. If, however, the tissue surrounding the nerve ending has been traumatised in some way, the nerve ending will be exposed to a range of chemical agents released from the damaged cells. There are many such inflammatory mediators released in this way and new ones are still being discovered

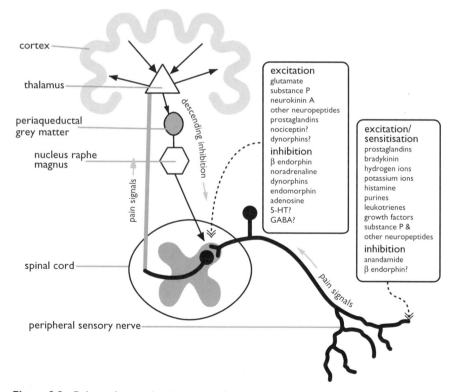

cortex

thalamus

periaqueductal grey matter

nucleus raphe magnus

descending inhibition

pain signals

spinal cord

peripheral sensory nerve

pain signals

excitation
glutamate
substance P
neurokinin A
other neuropeptides
prostaglandins
nociceptin?
dynorphins?

inhibition
β endorphin
noradrenaline
dynorphins
endomorphin
adenosine
5-HT?
GABA?

excitation/ sensitisation
prostaglandins
bradykinin
hydrogen ions
potassium ions
histamine
purines
leukotrienes
growth factors
substance P & other neuropeptides

inhibition
anandamide
β endorphin?

Figure 2.2 Pain pathways. A wide variety of substances can increase or decrease the frequency of firing in neurones carrying pain signals. This is particularly important at the level of the spinal cord, where the signal is 'gated'; however, 'gating' probably occurs at several different levels, especially at the thalamus. The higher up the CNS the signal goes, the more complex the processing becomes and the less certain is our knowledge of what is happening.

(Fig. 2.2). Some of these agents may have more than one action; for instance they may be involved in tissue repair or acting on other cells and their effects on sensory nerve endings may be incidental. More importantly, the constituents of the mix may be relevant in the effect on the nerve endings, and different traumas to different cells may produce different chemicals and hence a range of responses.

While some of these agents released may cause a direct excitation of the nerve ending, others may increase the sensitivity of the nerve endings to subsequent noxious stimuli or to other components of the 'inflammatory soup'. This may also render stimuli previously perceived as innocuous, for instance gentle pressure on the skin, to be perceived as noxious. This altered sensation is termed 'allodynia'.

Spinal cord

The impulses in sensory fibres make their first synapse at the level of the dorsal horn of the grey matter of the spinal cord. This is the first major site where chemical neurotransmitter agents are involved in the propagation of ongoing impulses and is thus important as a site of drug action.

After synapsing within the superficial layers of the dorsal horn the noxious signal is carried forward to the brain on the contralateral side, mainly in the spinothalamic and spinoreticular tracts. However, synapses within the grey matter of the spinal cord also connect with other areas, including the ventral horn, to make up the 'reflex arc' and produce a simple motor withdrawal response; synapses in other regions of the spinal cord may produce a variety of responses, such as local cardiovascular effects. If lesions occur within these neurones in the spinal cord or higher levels in the brain, then aberrant pain perception may occur in the absence of noxious stimuli.

One of the best described intrinsic control mechanisms occurs in afferent pain transmission at the level of the spinal cord. This is the 'gate theory' as first proposed by Melzack and Wall in 1965 which proposed that the signal passed up to the brain is a summation of the excitatory and inhibitory inputs (Fig. 2.2). Much of the basic concept of gate control has stood the test of time, but as with almost all things in biological systems, reality is somewhat more complicated than was first thought. There are almost certainly two levels of gating within the spinal cord, one at the level of entry to the dorsal horn and another at the level of the afferent input to the ascending dorsal columns (Wall 1992). Other sites of control may well exist at a variety of levels, for example acupuncture analgesia is thought to be mediated by A fibre input stimulating inhibitory interneurons which then reduce nociceptive signals in the transmission neurones. The purpose of this mechanism may be to prevent the animal being totally overwhelmed by a particularly intense pain and thereby facilitating survival by allowing some form of escape behaviour.

Central connections

After the afferent fibres enter the brain they again synapse at a variety of levels, of which the thalamus is thought to be most important (Fig. 2.2). The most rostral area involved in pain control is the prefrontal cortex (also involved in cognition) or medial frontal cortex, but other areas of the cortex are presumably involved in pain perception. It is interesting to speculate at which level a noxious stimulus actually becomes perceived as pain. Some have suggested the level of the thalamus, while others propose that it is a purely cortical effect.

Some of the ascending fibres terminate in the reticular formation, which is thought to govern consciousness and level of sleep. A practical consequence of this is that increased reticular activity produced by increased noxious input can overcome the effects of general anaesthetics.

There are a variety of other pathways from the spinal cord to different parts of the brain, but their importance has not been studied. There are also likely to be species differences in these pathways, which may account for the apparent varying responses to similar potential painful conditions in different species.

Descending control

The demonstration that electrical stimulation of particular regions of the brain could produce analgesia (Reynolds 1969, Meyer & Liebskind 1974) led to the concept that animals had an intrinsic pain control system which produced a descending inhibition of pain perception. This concept has allowed not only a much better understanding of the action of analgesic drugs but also an improved understanding of how pain perception is modulated internally. Two of the key areas in the brain which can be demonstrated to be integrating centres for descending inhibition are the periaqueductal grey area in the midbrain and the ventromedial medulla (Basbaum & Fields 1984, Fields & Besson 1988).

The descending control system exerts its effects at a variety of levels including the midbrain, the medulla and, particularly, the spinal cord. All of these effects act to reduce or modulate the ascending noxious information and hence to reduce the sensation of pain at the levels of perception. An interesting example of this is the situation where a racehorse can fracture various bones but not go lame until the excitement of the race is over. Also of interest for the pharmacological approach to pain control is the wide range of neurotransmitter agents involved in the synapses between these centres, including glutamate, noradrenaline, 5-hydroxytryptamine (5-HT, serotonin), γ-aminobutyric acid (GABA) and endogenous opioid peptides. Recently it has been suggested that agents such as adenosine and prostacyclin might be involved in nociceptive processing.

What is the purpose of such a system? We have a sophisticated system for detecting a range of noxious or potentially damaging stimuli. A further system whereby locally released agents can amplify or augment the sensitivity of this system is present. Finally, an additional complicated arrangement of neurones is superimposed on these to reduce the input from the receptor system. We assume that this system is arranged to protect the organism from external noxious agents. Further augmenting processes are included to prevent the organism from ignoring these agents, i.e. the system can become sensitised if some damage occurs. However, there could be situations, detected and assessed by higher centres, whereby the survival of the animal is best served by ignoring or down-grading the input from the noxious stimuli, e.g. to run away from the immediate danger of predation. Similarly, if some damage has occurred and the animal has responded to escape from the damaging agent, then the animal's survival might best be served by not responding further to the pain, but by getting on with finding food or a mate, for instance.

Central sensitisation

Sensitisation can occur in the central nervous system as well as peripheral sites. This is an interesting example of plasticity, i.e. the 'pain' signal changes over time. The original concept of a central nervous system was similar to a biological computer, namely a series of integrating parts connected by a system of wires. Recovery in damaged areas was presumed to take place by information being re-routed through existing pathways and by preexisting integrating areas assuming additional duties. These views were supported by the inability of mature neurones to divide, and the failure to replace killed or expired neurones by neighbouring neurones. Such a process is seen in progressive neurological disorders such as Parkinsonism, where the gradual loss and failure to replace the dopaminergic neurones of the substantia nigra leads to a remorseless progression of the motor disorders of this disease. Yet it has always been obvious that functional changes do take place within the brain. For instance, the mature brain is capable of many additional functions compared to the immature brain, and one of the most obvious areas is learning and memory. Many studies have now suggested that these are processes which take place within the neurones, and they involve neurochemical events similar to those seen in synaptic transmission processes, involving ionic movements across cell membranes and neurotransmitters such as glutamate. Plasticity can also occur by 'rewiring'. A variety of chemicals, e.g. nerve growth factor, oestrogen, and some cytokines can cause neurones to grow sprouts which then form new synapses. These chemicals are probably released during injury and even during abnormal neuronal activity of the type that gives rise to pain.

Studies (e.g. Woolf & Chong 1993) now indicate that pain also can cause changes in brain and spinal cord neurones that result in a heightened perception of pain after a period of stimulation (hyperalgesia). It is interesting to note that this central sensitisation was first proposed by a group of clinicians using data based on empirical observations of postoperative pain experienced by patients

(McQuay et al 1988). The demonstration of clear effects in human patients was not easy, due to both the multiplicity of drugs used (e.g. premedicants, muscle relaxants, cardiovascular agents and anaesthetics) and the inability to have untreated controls, not to mention the high level of placebo effects seen in man. However, despite some initial scepticism, the acceptance of central sensitisation to pain, and the fact that it is easier to prevent it using analgesic drugs given before the pain starts (pre-emptive analgesia) than to treat the subsequent hyper-algesia, now seems to be well established (Lascelles et al 1994, 1995).

The physiological mechanism of central sensitisation is complex and occurs within both the spinal cord and brain. Glutamate, acting at the N-methyl-D-aspartate (NMDA) receptor, is probably the main transmitter involved. The NMDA receptor is initially blocked by a magnesium ion; when glutamate causes depolarisation of a neurone by an action at the amino methylisoxazole proprionic acid (AMPA) receptor (the main process involved in normal fast transmission across a synapse), this magnesium ion is displaced so the next packet of gluta-mate causes both the AMPA and NMDA receptors to open and the cell is more likely to fire. This is thought to be an important process in central sensitisation to both pain and memory. There is increasing evidence that metabotropic gluta-mate receptors are also involved in amplifying the signal at this level. Other transmitters such as tachykinins (particularly substance P) are also involved. Early onset genes such as *c-fos* are activated and this will cause RNA changes that could result in increased peptide transmitter synthesis or changed receptor syn-thesis, or even growth factor production. Changes in enkephalins and pre-

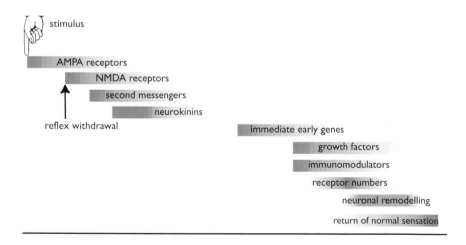

Figure 2.3 Processes involved in pain plasticity. The different mechanisms involved in pain sensation ensure that the pain will vary in nature and intensity with time. The processes involved and the time to resolution and restoration of normal sensation usually depend on the nature of the injury. In man, and probably also in animals, pain can persist beyond healing of the injury, presumably by some of these processes failing to return to normal.

enkephalins have been observed in areas of the spinal cord and are associated with a specific pain stimulus as well as changes in early onset genes (Noguchi et al 1992). These changes have been seen to take place within minutes and hours of a pain stimulus (Woolf and Chong 1993). It is interesting that an endogenous peptide with a very similar structure to the enkephalins (nociceptin) has been reported to cause pain in rats. The temporal spectrum of changes associated with pain perception can range from milliseconds to months, years and even for life in the case of memory, learning or neural damage (Fig. 2.3).

Other physiological responses

The motor response to a noxious stimulus, the 'reflex arc', has already been referred to, and even at this relatively simple level, it is obvious that there are control mechanisms since the withdrawal only occurs once, although the pain may well continue. However, there are many other physiological responses which occur after a noxious stimulus which may not have the obvious relevance that the reflex arc does. The autonomic reflexes are well documented and include such things as heart rate and blood pressure changes, alterations to respiratory rate and pattern, sweating, piloerection, gut motility and many others. However, these are unreliable indicators of pain although they are often used in animals as markers for pain intensity and analgesic efficacy. All of the changes listed can be induced or modified by stress-related endocrine activity, drugs or external physical effects, and to use them as sole indicators of the presence or otherwise of pain is very unwise (see chapter 4).

Similarly, pain or injury can cause profound endocrine changes and release of hormones from the pituitary, thyroid, parathyroid and adrenal glands and possibly other endocrine organs as well. Like the autonomic reflexes, these responses can be very unreliable indicators of pain although they are commonly used as such in animal studies. Many of the hormones in the body are released in a pulsatile manner and circulating levels can vary enormously over a short period; consequently, recorded levels are often very unreliable indicators of actual hormone release. However, the most important factor is that the endocrine changes can be influenced by many different inputs other than pain. In people, the levels of stress hormones in witnesses to an accident can be higher than those of the victim, and we know that in several species, isolation in unusual surroundings can produce greater changes in stress hormones, such as cortisol, than quite significant noxious stimuli (Parrot et al 1987). In chronic pain (and thus stress) the levels of circulating stress hormones are actually reduced (Ley et al 1991).

Behavioural changes

Although they may not obviously fall into a discussion on 'physiology of pain,' behavioural changes can be considered as the 'overall integrated physiological response' to pain and as such are worthy of consideration here. Since they constitute an *integrated* response, they are obviously complex, difficult to interpret and difficult to quantify, but for pain evaluation in animals, they are perhaps the most useful observation. It is important to realise that alteration of behavioural changes with drugs is not the same thing as analgesia. This is particularly relevant with the sedative drugs which can have a profound effect on behaviour without altering pain perception.

Again, there are many problems: different location of pains will cause different behaviours; different intensities of pain and different environments will also influence response; responses will vary between different animal species. Clearly, chronic pain, intermittent pain and acute pain will produce different responses, and perhaps most difficult of all, different individuals will respond differently to an identical stimulus. When assessing behavioural values, it is important to remember that not all behaviours will have the same 'weight' as indicators of pain (this particularly applies to those associated with autonomic control, as indicated earlier). Very often the most complex behaviour will be the most significant; for instance, if a dog bares its teeth as you move your hand towards a particular leg, that is probably a stronger indicator than panting or heart rate, and should be assessed as such (see chapter 4).

Probably the most widely studied species in terms of behaviour when in pain is, of course, man, and although we must exercise great care in transposing theories across species, there are some aspects of human pain behaviour which should cause us some concern when dealing with animals. The first of these concerns is the not infrequent incidence of pain without any apparent pathology. It is accepted in these situations that the perception of pain is real, that the patients are not suffering from delusions resulting from a psychological disorder, and that in many cases therapy in some form, often of a type other than conventional analgesics, can give lasting relief. Would a similar situation account for animals which display erratic or vicious behaviour, and how often would non-lesion pain be considered as a differential diagnosis? The other human phenomenon which has a fascination of its own, and is in some ways a corollary of non-lesion pain, is placebo analgesia.

A clear placebo effect is demonstrable in pain therapy in humans – so much so that some clinicians have seriously suggested that primary therapy for some chronic pain conditions should always be placebo, since the recovery rate is often as high as 20% without exposing the patient to the risks of drug therapy. After this the clinician can then address the non-responders to placebo with appropriate analgesics, in some cases with about the same expectation of success! Should we consider if animals can show placebo responses? We know that most of the physiological and pathological responses to noxious input is the same in humans and animals, the pathways and the neurotransmitters are the same, many of the autonomic and endocrine responses are the same and the same analgesics seem to reduce pain symptoms and behaviours at similar doses when adjusted for wide weight ranges. Perhaps the placebo response would be the same? The fascinating role of the subjective aspects of pain in animals is likely to become more important as our knowledge of this area advances from witchcraft to science.

In conclusion, knowledge of the physiological processes associated with pain helps obtain the correct diagnosis, helps some assessment of the intensity and helps consider the prognosis in many situations. In addition, it facilitates the rational and appropriate usage of anaesthetic and analgesic drugs and allows evaluation of the efficacy of those agents in each particular case. It also allows the usage of these agents to effect, rather than relying on simple dosage rates, which may only be effective in a proportion of cases.

References

Basbaum, A. and Fields, H.L. (1984) Endogenous pain control systems: brain stem spinal pathways and endorphin circuitry. *Annual Review of Neuroscience* **7**: 309–338.

Fields, H.L. and Besson, J.M. (eds) (1988) Descending brainstem controls of nociceptive transmission. *Progress in Brain Research* **77**: Elsevier, Amsterdam.

Lascelles, B.D.X., Waterman, A.E., Henderson, G. and Livingston, A. (1994) Central sensitization as a result of surgical pain – the value of pre-emptive analgesia. *Proceedings of the 5th International Congress on Veterinary Anaesthesia*, p 159.

Lascelles, B.D.X., Waterman, A.E., Cripps, P.J., Livingston, A. and Henderson, G. (1995) Central sensitization as result of surgical pain: investigation of the pre-emptive value of pethidine for ovariohysterectomy in the rat. *Pain*, **62**: 201–212.

Ley, S.J., Livingston, A. and Waterman, A.E. (1991) The effects of clinically occurring chronic lameness in sheep on the concentration of plasma cortisol, prolactin and vasopressin. *Veterinary Record* **129**: 45–47.

McQuay, H.J., Carroll, D. and Moore, R.A. (1988) Post-operative orthopaedic pain – the effect of opiate premedication and local anaesthetic blocks. *Pain* **33**: 291 295.

Melzack, R. and Wall, P.D. (1965) Pain mechanisms: a new theory. *Science* **150**: 971–979.

Meyer, D.J. and Liebskind, J.C. (1974) Pain reduction by focal electrical stimulation of the brain: an anatomical and behavioural analysis. *Brain Research* **68**: 73–93.

Noguchi, K., Dubner, R. and Ruda, M.A. (1992) Preproenkephalin mRNA in spinal dorsal horn neurones is induced by peripheral inflammation and is co-localised with fos and fos related proteins. *Neuroscience* **46**: 561–570.

Parrot, R.F., Thornton, S.N., Forsling, M.L. and Delaney, C.E. (1987) Endocrine and behavioural factors affecting water balance in sheep subjected to isolation stress. *Journal of Endocrinology* **112**: 305–310.

Reynolds, D.V. (1969) Surgery in the rat during electrical analgesia induced by focal brain stimulation. *Science* **164**: 444–445.

Wall, P.D. (1992) Defining 'pain' in animals. In: Short, C.E. and Van Poznak, A. (eds) *Animal Pain*. Churchill Livingstone, New York, pp 63–79.

Woolf, C.J. and Chong, M.S. (1993) Pre-emptive analgesia; treating post-operative pain by preventing the establishment of central sensitization. *Anesthesia and Analgesia* **77**: 293–299.

PHARMACOLOGY OF ANALGESIC DRUGS

3

A.M. Nolan

With a knowledge of the major pain pathways (chapter 2), the mediators involved in relaying pain information, the mediators involved in inflammation and the consequences of inflammation to the animal in terms of altered pain processing, it is possible to understand the use of drugs to alleviate pain. Analgesics are usually considered to be drugs which abolish pain. This is probably too simplistic a view of their function since they may differentially affect the sensory and the affective components of pain. Some drugs used for the control of pain may be antihyperalgesic rather than analgesic, i.e. they restore reduced pain thresholds (see chapter 2) to normal (e.g. non-steroidal antiinflammatory drugs), rather than elevating pain thresholds (e.g. local anaesthetic drugs). Most analgesic drugs are hypoalgesic, i.e. they reduce pain rather than abolish it, although this feature is generally dose dependent.

Analgesic drugs may be divided into five main classes:

1. Opioids
2. Non-steroidal antiinflammatory drugs (NSAIDs)
3. Local anaesthetics
4. Alpha-2 adrenoceptor agonists
5. Miscellaneous drugs, e.g. ketamine, nitrous oxide.

Drugs such as corticosteroids may also be useful by virtue of their antiinflammatory activity, while many other classes of drugs have been shown to modify pain information processing in experimental studies (e.g. the neurokinin 1 antagonists) but are not yet available for clinical use.

Opioids

Opioid drugs have been used for the relief of pain for over 2000 years and today they are still of enormous therapeutic importance as the drugs of choice for the treatment of moderate to severe pain. Indeed, in current medical and veterinary practice, morphine remains the mainstay therapy for severe pain. The term 'opiate' describes drugs derived from opium such as morphine, first isolated in 1806, and codeine. With the development of synthetic analogues of these drugs, the term 'opioid' was introduced to represent all drugs that act in a similar manner to morphine. The opioid analgesics may be referred to as narcotic

	Receptor		
	μ	κ	δ
Morphine	+++	+/–	+/–
Pethidine	++	+/–	–
Fentanyl	+++	–	–
Alfentanil	+++	–	–
Etorphine	+++	++	++
Buprenorphine	+++	++	+/–
Butorphanol	++	++	–
Naloxone	+++	+	+

Table 3.1 Selectivity of opioid drugs used in animals.

analgesics because of their ability to induce narcosis, a state of drowsiness, in humans and in some animal species. Opioids have been used in veterinary medicine for many purposes, and with an increasing recognition of the adverse effects of pain in animals over the past 10 years, their frequency of use to attenuate pain has grown.

The identification of opioid binding sites in mammalian brain tissue in the 1970s was a watershed in the understanding of how opioid drugs act to produce their effects (Goldstein et al 1971, Pert & Snyder 1973). Opioids act on at least three different opioid receptors: mu (μ), kappa (κ) and delta (δ) receptors (Table 3.1). These receptors have been reclassified as OP_3 (μ), OP_2 (κ) and OP_1 (δ), in accordance with the chronological sequence of cloning the receptors. The sigma receptor, originally identified as an opioid receptor, is not now considered to fit the required criteria. The existence of the epsilon (ε) receptor, postulated as the binding site for the endogenous opioid β endorphin, is controversial. Recent work in the 1990s has indicated the existence of a new orphan opioid receptor, an opioid-like receptor with considerable homology to other opioid receptors, termed ORL1 (Fukuda et al 1994). Pharmacological studies have suggested the existence of μ receptor subtypes, μ1 and μ2, κ receptor subtypes ($κ_1$, $κ_2$, $κ_3$) and multiple δ opioid receptors (δ1, δ2); however, to date, these have not been supported by cloning experiments. The possibility of alternative splicing mechanisms of the receptor genes giving rise to receptor subtypes with altered functional responses exists (Zaki et al 1996). The opioid receptors are activated by a family of structurally related endogenous petides. Genes encoding three families of opioid peptides, proenkephalin, prodynorphin and pro-opiomelanocortin have been cloned.

The distribution of opioid receptors has been described in detail in many animal species (Atweh & Kuhar 1977 a, b, c; Wamsley et al 1982). Each receptor is distributed differently throughout the CNS. High densities of opioid receptors are found in areas of the central nervous system (CNS) associated with the processing of nociceptive information in all species studied. Opioid receptors are also found throughout the periphery and here they mediate opioid effects such as decreasing gastrointestinal motility. While species similarities are undoubtedly present, it cannot be assumed directly that a certain receptor subtype will have an identical function in all species. For example, drugs active primarily at μ receptor sites cause mild narcosis in humans but increase locomotor activity in the horse (Combie et al 1981, Nolan et al 1994).

Endogenous opioids such as metenkephalin, leuenkephalin, the dynorphins, β endorphin, and others, have been demonstrated in areas of the CNS concerned with the processing of nociceptive information, and these peptides act at one or more of the opioid receptors. Nociceptin/orphanin FQ, a peptide first isolated in 1995 from rat and pig brains, is the endogenous ligand for the orphan opioid receptor (Meunier et al 1995). While the precise physiological roles of these and other neuropeptides in pain processing remain to be elucidated, there is evidence that opioid peptides such as metenkephalin may regulate, in either a positive or negative manner, the release of other neuropeptides which transmit noxious information from the periphery to the spinal cord. In the brain, these peptides are also associated with other functions such as learning and memory.

Knowledge of the molecular biology of the opioid receptors (for review see Minami & Satoh 1995) and their endogenous ligands has enabled scientists to create animal models in which specific genes have been deleted, altered or replaced. Mice lacking the β endorphin gene show normal analgesia to morphine but do not exhibit opioid stress-induced analgesia when challenged with a stress situation, while mice lacking the μ receptor display no analgesia to morphine but retain analgesia to κ agonists. The role of many of the endogenous opioids and their receptors may thus be characterised further in the near future.

The three major subtypes of opioid receptor act on recognised effector systems to cause a cellular effect. Opioid receptors are coupled via guanine triphosphate (GTP)-binding proteins to adenylate cyclase and alter its activity, generally inducing inhibition of the enzyme. Opioid receptor activation also causes inhibition of voltage-dependent calcium channels, via G proteins. Opioids may induce membrane hyperpolarisation by increasing potassium conductance, an effect mediated via G proteins, and there is evidence that opioids mobilise calcium from intracellular stores as a consequence of phospholipase C activation.

Opioid drugs may be classified according to their receptor selectivity and may be active at one, two or all of the receptors. The differences in drug receptor selectivity confer discrete properties on individual drugs and will help predict the pharmacological properties of a given drug in an individual animal species. Activation of a receptor subtype is associated with a particular pharmacological profile; for example, μ selective agonists induce euphoria in humans, while κ selective drugs induce dysphoria. In general, the most effective analgesic drugs in clinical use act selectively at μ receptors. These include morphine, pethidine, fentanyl, alfentanil and buprenorphine. Butorphanol is active at μ receptors but also has significant activity at κ receptors (Garner et al 1997).

23

Opioids are also categorised as either agonists, partial agonists, mixed agonist-antagonists, or antagonists, which describes their ability to induce a response once bound to a receptor. Agonists can induce a maximal response while partial agonists cannot induce a maximal response irrespective of the dose administered. Antagonists bind to receptors but produce no response. Drugs may be agonists at one receptor subtype while displaying antagonist or partial agonist activity at another.

Actions of opioids

Analgesia

Opioids produce analgesia by binding to either μ, κ or δ receptors located within the CNS, either spinally or supraspinally, although recently the suggestion that opioid analgesia can be brought about by activation of opioid receptors located peripherally in inflamed tissues has gained more acceptance (Stein 1993). All opioid drugs displaying agonist activity at μ receptors are analgesics. The degree of analgesia produced will depend on whether the drug is an agonist or a partial agonist, on the dose administered and on the pharmacokinetics of the drugs in a given species. It is unwise to extrapolate clinical data from humans to determine dosage regimes for animals, since the pharmacokinetics of drugs vary considerably between species. Most of the opioids commonly used in veterinary medicine belong to the μ selective group, e.g. morphine, pethidine, fentanyl, oxymorphone, methadone, buprenorphine (partial agonist) and butorphanol (partial agonist with significant κ activity). Opioids with selective κ activity have not been developed for use in humans due to the dysphoria which accompanies these drugs. Recently, there has been interest in the development of δ opioid agonists/partial agonists since these drugs may have fewer side-effects than μ selective agents. Opioids reduce the sensation of pain and in humans they appear to reduce the psychological stress associated with pain. They may have a pre-emptive effect (see chapter 5) when used before the onset of tissue damage. A pre-emptive effect has been shown in the immediate postoperative period in dogs for pethidine, and in rodents, but is controversial in humans.

Studies in animals have shown that local injection of low doses of opioids into an area of inflammation produces analgesia; thus it appears that opioid receptors are involved in the mediation of analgesic effects in the periphery. Opioid receptors are present on peripheral nerve endings and on inflammatory cells. Peripheral analgesic opioid effects are not obvious in normal tissues but become apparent within a short period after the start of inflammation. Clinical studies in humans have examined the efficacy of intra-articular administration of morphine into the knee joint of patients undergoing orthopaedic surgery, and the majority of studies published have reported analgesia from low doses of morphine (0.5–6 mg total dose), similar in intensity to that recorded with local anaesthetics, which is long-lasting (up to 48 h) (Joshi et al 1993, Heine et al

1994). No side-effects have been reported. There have been few reports to date regarding the use and efficacy of local opioid administration in animals following orthopaedic surgery, although they may be useful, particularly in combination with local anaesthetic agents.

Respiratory depression

Opioid drugs cause respiratory depression by decreasing the responsiveness of the respiratory centre to carbon dioxide (Florez et al 1968); the hypoxic stimulus to breathing is unaffected. Opioids may alter respiratory rate, rhythmicity and pattern, and minute volume. Respiratory rate alone is not a reliable index of opioid-induced depression since apparently adequate respiratory rates may be recorded in the presence of elevated arterial carbon dioxide tensions. In general, breathing rate is slowed but tidal volume is unaffected, although dogs in particular may pant following administration of high doses. Respiratory depression, while a concern for medical colleagues using opioids in humans, does not appear to be a problem in animals and clinical reports of significant opioid induced respiratory depression are rare. The potent opioids fentanyl and alfentanil used in animals intraoperatively to provide profound analgesia do cause respiratory depression which generally requires that the animal be ventilated (Nolan & Reid 1991).

Cardiovascular effects

The effects of opioid drugs on the cardiovascular system are very variable depending on the species, the drug, the route of administration and the type of preparation. Morphine and related drugs cause centrally-mediated bradycardia and hypotension, although the degree of hypotension is mild (Martin 1983). These effects are related to their action on opioid receptors located in the brainstem, causing inhibition of sympathetic tone to the heart. The bradycardia associated with intravenous administration of the potent opioids fentanyl and alfentanil can be severe but is inhibited/attenuated by administration of an antimuscarinic drug such as atropine (Nolan & Reid 1991). Pethidine causes hypotension if injected i.v., probably due to histamine release. When given i.v., occasionally morphine may induce histamine release which can cause hypotension and, on very rare occasions, bronchospasm. The amount of histamine released is related to the total dose and the rate of injection; thus slow injection intravenously is normally safe. Low doses of morphine have been used without adverse cardiovascular effects in horses during halothane anaesthesia (Nolan et al 1991). Most opioids have little effect on myocardial contractility, but pethidine at clinically relevant doses in dogs (3–5 mg/kg) induces a decrease in contractility which can become significant at higher doses (Freye 1974).

25

The opioid etorphine has significant cardiovascular effects in some species (Lees & Hillidge 1976). Hypertension and tachycardia are observed following injection of the etorphine–acepromazine combination ('large animal immobilon') in horses with pronounced decreases in stroke index (Lees & Hillidge 1975). Cardiovascular effects of the etorphine–methotrimeprazine ('small animal immobilon') combination in dogs include hypotension and bradycardia (Schlarmann et al 1973).

Antitussive activity

Opioids such as codeine and morphine are well known antitussive drugs. Drugs active at μ and κ sites are effective antitussive agents, while it appears that δ opioid receptors play only a minor role in mediating these effects (Bolser 1996). There is a poor association between the antitussive effects of opioid drugs and their analgesic properties; thus codeine has antitussive activity at subanalgesic doses, while pholcodine is even more potent as an antitussive agent. Butorphanol was originally licensed for use in dogs as an antitussive agent.

Mood-altering properties

Opioids active at the μ receptor generally induce euphoria in humans although unpleasant mood alterations have been described (Walker & Zacny 1999) and appear to produce similar positive reinforcement behaviours in animals, while κ receptor activation is associated with dysphoria in humans and work carried out in laboratory animals would suggest that treatment with κ receptor drugs is highly aversive (Pfeiffer 1990, Simonin et al 1998). Butorphanol given alone induces a stress response in dogs which has been attributed to dysphasia (Fox et al 1998).

Effects on gastrointestinal motility

Opioids reduce the propulsive activity of the gastrointestinal tract (Kromer 1988). Smooth muscle and sphincter tone tend to be increased, but peristalsis is decreased. Morphine induces vomiting by activating the chemoreceptor trigger zone, but appears to be the only opioid which induces vomiting in dogs and cats. Other opioids produce this effect in humans along with nausea. Butorphanol has shown specific antiemetic activity in humans and in dogs (Moore et al 1994) and does not cause vomiting in animals (nor does buprenorphine). Pethidine has a spasmolytic action on the gut due to its anticholinergic activity (Hustveit & Setekleiv 1993).

Locomotor activity

Opioids induce a decrease in spontaneous motor activity in some species, e.g. in humans, and also in dogs depending on the drug and dose. In general, decreased motor activity is also observed in cats when clinically relevant doses are used. Reports of maniacal excitement in this species relate to the use of morphine at very high doses (100 times greater than the clinical dose). Horses show increased locomotor activity when given opioid drugs, and other behaviours such as compulsive eating behaviour and agitation (Combie et al 1981, Nolan et al 1994). Many of these effects are reduced when opioids are used in combination with the tranquilliser acepromazine or the alpha-2 adrenoceptor agonist sedatives such as xylazine (Nolan & Hall 1984).

Tolerance and dependence

Tolerance can be defined as the decrease in effectiveness of a drug after repeated administration. It is a complex phenomenon with important therapeutic implications where drugs are to be administered over a prolonged period of time. While this occurs frequently in humans, it is rare for opioids to be used therapeutically for longer than 4–5 days in any animal species. Physical dependence is the need to continue administration of a drug following prior exposure in order to prevent the development of an abstinence syndrome. There have been no reports of this occurring clinically in animals, which is likely to be a reflection of the short-term clinical use of opioids in animals.

The phenomenon of dependence is significant for veterinary practitioners as it has implications for the storing and prescribing of opioid drugs. Most opioids are subject to control under the Misuse of Drugs Act 1971, either under Schedule 2 or Schedule 3 (see below). Butorphanol is an exception, although it is now subjected to control in the USA, presumably due to its relatively poor ability to induce dependence. However, there is some evidence in laboratory animals that a substantial degree of physical dependence may be induced by butorphanol (Horan & Ho 1991).

Other effects

Opioids are given to animals before surgery in order to reduce the amount of anaesthetic agent required. In cats, dogs (e.g. Michelsen et al 1996, Ilkiw et al 1997) and other species (Steffey et al 1994, Concannon et al 1995), opioids are effective in this respect. However, some studies in horses have indicated that use of opioids preoperatively and intraoperatively does not reduce the concentration of inhalational anaesthetic required to maintain anaesthesia (Matthews & Lindsay 1990). This may be a function of the test system used to determine the inhalational anaesthetic requirements in experimental studies, since opioids induce sleep-like electroencephalogram patterns in horses similar to those patterns recorded in other species (Johnson & Taylor 1997). Low doses of the opioids morphine and butorphanol given intravenously to horses during anaesthesia had minimal effects on respiration or on cardiovascular function (Nolan et al 1988).

Endogenous opioids as well as catecholamines, ACTH and glucocorticoids are important in the neurochemical mechanisms of stress. For many years it has been recognised that stress induces analgesia both in experimental animals and in clinical patients. The endogenous opioid systems are widely represented in central and peripheral regions which are involved in the stress response: the hypothalamus, the pituitary gland and the adrenal glands. Endogenous opioid systems are not usually tonically active; thus opioid antagonists have little or no effect in the resting state. However, when animals encounter stressful situations, endogenous opioids are released which may help in developing adaptive strategies. Opioid drugs and opioid peptides may alter the production of adrenocortical steroids in animals (Kapas et al 1995).

Pharmacokinetics and metabolism

The pharmacokinetics of opioid drugs have not been comprehensively described in most animal species, with the exception of pethidine in the dog and alfentanil and fentanyl in several species. In general, opioids are well absorbed from the gut but due to a high first-pass metabolism effect, are only poorly bioavailable when given orally. They are generally well absorbed from intramuscular and subcutaneous routes (provided the animal has good tissue perfusion), and they are generally highly metabolised by the liver (glucuronidation, demethylation, etc.). Some metabolites have analgesic activity, e.g. morphine-6-glucuronide. Morphine is extensively conjugated with glucuronic acid and this hepatic pathway accounts for approx. 50% of morphine metabolism in anaesthetised dogs (Jacqz et al 1986); extrahepatic metabolism of morphine accounts for the other 50%. While renal metabolism of morphine occurs in humans, this does not appear to be the case in dogs. Fentanyl is cleared by lung tissue. Fentanyl and alfentanil undergo either dealkylation or demethylation followed by amide hydrolysis and the metabolites are then excreted primarily in the urine. Buprenorphine is extensively metabolised in dogs, with only 1% unchanged buprenorphine appearing in the urine and bile. The main metabolite is buprenorphine glucuronide which is excreted in bile (see below). Remifentanil, an ultra short-acting opioid recently developed for use by infusion in humans, is metabolised by plasma esterases (Peacock & Frances 1997). The pharmacokinetics of remifentanil in dogs would suggest that it may be useful, as part of a balanced anaesthetic technique (see below).

Specific pharmacological features of individual drugs

Morphine

In spite of its widespread use over many years in animals, data on the clinical pharmacology of morphine in animals are not comprehensive. Morphine is widely distributed throughout the body, is rapidly cleared and has a relatively short elimination half-life (1–2 h) (Merrell et al 1990). The drug is almost completely absorbed when administered intramuscularly. The rapid clearance of morphine and the short elimination half-life suggest that the regime of administering morphine approximately every 4 h in dogs may be inappropriate. However, morphine persists in the cerebrospinal fluid much longer than in plasma and this may be a more accurate reflection of the duration of action of analgesia. Cats do not metabolise morphine as rapidly as other species and in these animals the dosing interval is extended (4–6 h). Morphine is most commonly used in small animals and although its use has been described in horses it is not frequently adopted in pain management protocols in this species. It frequently induces vomiting when given to conscious dogs before surgery; however, this side-effect is seldom observed when morphine is used postoperatively or in animals suffering from acute trauma. Morphine, like all the opioids, is not licensed for use in animals intended for human consumption. It appears to be analgesic in cattle and pigs, but the duration of action is probably considerably less than 4 h due to more rapid metabolism. For dosing information see chapter 5. When given by oral or rectal routes, the bioavailability of morphine in dogs is low (Barnhart et al 2000).

Papaveretum is a crude form of morphine licensed in humans as a combination product along with other alkaloids. Its actions are very similar to those of morphine.

Pethidine

Pethidine is less potent than morphine. It, too, is rapidly cleared from the body (Waterman & Kalthum 1989, 1990), particularly in the large animal species (Nolan et al 1988). It has a short duration of action in the treatment of surgical pain in dogs and cats, c. 2 h depending on the dose, while a duration of action less than 30 min appears to follow treatment of horses and ruminants. It is used frequently as part of a premedicant regime as it does not induce vomiting. It has a short onset time following i.m. injection and is useful in the management of acute trauma pain and surgical pain in dogs and cats. However, its short duration of action can be a disadvantage in managing pain after moderate to severe surgical procedures. Its anticholinergic activity is useful in the therapy of spasmodic colic in horses. For dosing information see chapter 5.

Fentanyl

Fentanyl is a highly potent opioid generally administered by bolus intravenous injection, by intermittent intravenous injection or by infusion. It is a selective μ opioid receptor agonist and is suitable as an intraoperative analgesic because of its short onset time, short duration of action and potency. It has a very large volume of distribution in dogs and has a high clearance value, but a relatively long elimination half-life. The elimination half-life is a reflection of the drug penetrating poorly perfused compartments such as fat, from which it is only slowly released. This widespread uptake by tissues throughout the body, a consequence of its high lipid solubility, limits the infusion time, since cumulation of the drug with long infusion periods (>2 h) is likely. Fentanyl has a rapid onset time, the peak effect being evident 2–5 min after i.v. injection (Waterman et al 1990, Nolan & Reid 1991). The duration of analgesic action is short, between 5–20 min depending on the dose given. It is a potent respiratory depressant, which generally limits its use in anaesthetised animals to those that are mechanically ventilated. It induces bradycardia, which may be obtunded by the use of an antimuscarinic drug. Muscle rigidity has been reported in humans with the use of high doses of fentanyl (Benthuysen & Stanley 1985); however, this effect is not common in animals, possibly due to the lower dose rates used.

Recently, fentanyl has been used in dogs and cats by the transdermal route (see below). Skin patches designed for use in humans containing fentanyl released at different dose rates (25, 50 µg/h) have been applied to dogs. These patches produced plasma fentanyl levels in dogs that were within the analgesic range recognised in humans after 24 h, although there is considerable inter-animal variation (Kyles et al 1996). Their use in humans is restricted to chronic pain therapy.

Fentanyl is available in a combination product along with the butyrophenone tranquilliser fluanisone, and is marketed as 'Hypnorm'. It is used as a neuroleptanaesthetic/neuroleptanalgesic mixture in rats, rabbits, mice and guinea pigs.

Fentanyl is also available in combination with droperidol in a propietary mixture ('Innovar': fentanyl, 0.4 mg/ml with droperidol, 20 mg/ml). It is used in dogs, cats, rabbits and laboratory rodents for premedication and sedation. It produces excellent analgesia of short duration (*c.* 30 min). However, the sedation persists for considerably longer.

Alfentanil

This drug is only administered by intravenous injection, either as a bolus or more commonly by intravenous infusion. The drug has a short elimination half-life (*c.* 0.4–2 h depending on the species), a small volume of distribution within the body and a moderately fast clearance (Pascoe et al 1991, Hoke et al 1997) and so is well suited to administration by infusion. Like fentanyl, alfentanil is a potent respiratory depressant and induces significant bradycardia at clinical doses; consequently it is recommended that animals are pretreated with an antimuscarinic drug such as atropine or glycopyrrolate before use. Its duration of action is very short (2–5 min). Alfentanil has also been used as a bolus before induction of anaesthesia with a barbiturate or propofol. It is most commonly used to provide intraoperative analgesia in small animals, given by intravenous infusion. When used in this manner it reduces the requirement for inhalational or intravenous anaesthetic drug maintenance (Ilkiw et al 1997), although this was not the case in horses (Pascoe et al 1993).

Sufentanil

Sufentanil is a thiamyl analogue of fentanyl with greater analgesic potency. It is used intravenously in humans as a bolus and by infusion, and is also given epidurally and intrathecally to provide spinal analgesia. The cardiovascular and respiratory effects are similar to those of fentanyl (Willens & Myslinski 1993). Its use by infusion in dogs with nitrous oxide has been described (Van Han et al 1996).

Remifentanil

(See New developments section on page 34.)

Buprenorphine

Buprenorphine is a potent μ selective partial opioid agonist which has a particularly high affinity for its receptor. The association of the drug with the receptor is slow and this is reflected in the slow onset time of action of the drug (30–60 min). Buprenorphine has a long elimination half-life in dogs, $c.$ 42 h, a large volume of distribution and moderately fast body clearance (Garrett & Chandran 1990). The slow terminal half-life of buprenorphine in dogs, probably a consequence of return of buprenorphine from a 'deep' tissue compartment such as fat, is not reflected in a particularly long duration of action (4–8 h). The elimination of buprenorphine is faster in sheep and the duration of action is shorter ($c.$ 3 h). Buprenorphine is given sublingually in humans, a route of administration which alows rapid absorption but by-passes the liver during the absorbative phase. However, this route is not practical in animals. Administration of the drug orally results in very poor bioavailability, between 3 and 6%. The actions of buprenorphine are not readily reversed with opioid antagonists. For dosing information see chapter 5.

Butorphanol

Butorphanol is a partial opioid agonist with activity at both μ and κ receptors. It was used in humans but unfavourable mood changes and variable analgesia resulted in limited use by the parenteral route. However, it is available as a nasal spray. Butorphanol is rapidly and almost completely absorbed after intramuscular or subcutaneous injection in dogs and reaches a peak plasma concentration within 30–45 min (Pfeffer et al 1980). The drug is lipophilic and is well distributed throughout the body, particularly in dogs and cows. Body clearance is high in dogs, cows and humans, but considerably slower in the horse. The elimination half-life was short in dogs, cows and horses (1–2 h), although even at low doses, butorphanol can be detected in cows milk for 36 h (Court et al 1992). The data suggest that if the therapeutic plasma concentration of butorphanol is the same in cows and horses, the dose required to produce analgesia may be higher in cows due to the greater volume of distribution. Analgesia is of short to moderate duration when butorphanol is used to control postoperative pain in dogs and cats (1–2.5 h), although data from experimental pain studies suggest a longer duration of action. The intensity of analgesia can be variable and its use is best restricted to animals in mild to moderate pain. Butorphanol appears to enhance considerably the tranquillising properties of acepromazine in animals. In the horse, butorphanol given alone induces an increase in locomotor activity (Nolan et al 1994), and it is most commonly used in this species in combination with sedatives or tranquillisers. Butorphanol is an effective antitussive agent and is licensed for this purpose in small animals. Licensed doses in the dogs and cat are lower than those suggested by experimental studies (Sawyer et al 1991).

Methadone

Methadone is a μ agonist which is similar in effect, but may have a longer duration of action, than morphine. It does not induce vomiting in dogs. It is commonly used in several European countries in combination with a tranquilliser such as acepromazine or a sedative such as medetomidine or xylazine, to produce deep sedation.

Naloxone

Naloxone is an opioid antagonist which is used in medical practice to antagonise the effects of full/partial agonists. It has a short duration of action, *c*. 30–60 min, and where it is used to antagonise side-effects of toxicity of opioid drugs in animals, clinicians must be prepared to repeat the dose at frequent intervals.

Epidural administration of opioid drugs

Opioid drugs can be applied directly onto the spinal cord. The upper layers of the dorsal horn grey matter contain high densities of opioid receptors, activation of which induces analgesia. In humans, direct delivery of the drug into the cerebrospinal fluid (intrathecal administration) is frequently employed, as is epidural injection; however, in animals epidural administration is most common. Morphine has been used in dogs, cats, horses and cattle and is probably the most useful opioid for epidural injection in veterinary medicine because of its long duration of action (Pascoe 1992) (see chapter 5). The main advantage over epidural local anaesthetic administration is that analgesia is induced without significant motor impairment. More lipid-soluble drugs, such as fentanyl, are shorter-acting and are not well retained within the CSF; they must be injected more often. Butorphanol has been used epidurally but it is not well retained within the CSF. The relatively less lipid-soluble morphine takes time to penetrate the spinal cord and the onset time is slow − *c.* 30–60 min to maximum effect; however, it is readily retained within the spinal cord tissue and the duration of action is long − from 12–24 h after a single administration. The apparently long duration of analgesic activity of morphine in humans has been explained by the relative persistence of morphine in the CSF. Segmental analgesia occurs following epidural morphine injection and spinal regions close to the site of injection exhibit more profound analgesia that is more rapid in onset than those further away.

The morphine used for epidural injection should be preservative-free, to avoid tissue damage, although some preservatives have been associated with no adverse side-effects (methylparaben, sodium metabisulphite). Side-effects of epidural morphine administration in humans include urinary retention, nausea, pruritis and, on occasions, delayed respiratory depression. Delayed respiratory depression is of particular concern in humans since it can occur many hours after morphine administration. Some side-effects are recognised in dogs: urinary retention on occasion and, not uncommonly, delayed hair regrowth around the site of epidural injection. Epidural morphine reduced the minimum alveolar concentration of halothane in dogs (Valverde et al 1989). As halothane is a cardiovascular depressant, adjunct therapy to reduce the requirement for halothane during anaesthesia and surgery, which in itself has minimal cardiovascular effect, must be regarded as advantageous.

Use of opioid analgesics

Opioids are used:
1. in the treatment of moderate to severe pain
2. as part of a neuroleptanalgesic technique
3. as part of a balanced anaesthetic technique to provide analgesia
4. as antitussives
5. to decrease gut motility.

More details of their clinical use are given in chapter 5.

Contraindications to the use of opioids

Where an animal is displaying respiratory depression, opioids are best avoided unless the animal is to be ventilated. Clearly, where respiratory depression is due to pain, e.g. fractured ribs, relief of pain will improve respiration. Many opioids increase intracranial pressure. This arises as a consequence of respiratory depression, which raises arterial carbon dioxide tension; elevated arterial carbon dioxide tension increases cerebral blood flow, which may raise intracranial pressure. Thus, in head injured patients, opioids are better avoided until a diagnosis is obtained and arterial carbon dioxide is regulated by controlled ventilation (see chapter 7). In animals with biliary obstruction or pancreatitis, morphine should be avoided as sphincter contraction can exacerbate the conditions. Pethidine, an opioid with spasmolytic activity, is a suitable alternative in these situations, although this opioid may not provide sufficient pain relief in these cases (see chapter 7).

New developments in opioid drug pharmacology

Transdermal fentanyl, i.e. application of fentanyl directly onto shaved skin, has been studied in dogs and cats. The high lipid solubility of the drug permits its absorption through the skin. Transdermal delivery systems for fentanyl have been developed for use in people and have been applied to animals (Kyles 1998). The transdermal skin patches consist of a drug reservoir containing fentanyl, an alcohol cellulose gel and a membrane which controls the rate of drug delivery to the skin. The patches that are available for use release fentanyl at differing rates (25, 50, 75 and 100 μg/h). Absorption is slow and it is recommended that patches are applied 20 h before the desired effect is required in dogs. Once peak plasma concentrations are achieved, the plasma concentration appears to remain relatively stable until the patch is removed. Studies in dogs have reported that using patches delivering fentanyl at 50 μg/h results in therapeutic plasma levels (>1 ng/ml) for prolonged periods. Patches were left on the skin for 72 h in dogs, whereas patches were left on cats for 104 h, with maintenance of plasma drug levels (Kyles et al 1996, Scherk-Nixon 1996). The decay of plasma levels after patch removal occurs over a period of up to 12 h. Problems with the patches include alteration in drug delivery/absorption rates with alterations in skin temperature and skin blood flow, failure of the patches to stay in place for a variety of reasons, and the potential for human abuse. Further work on their use is required before they can be recommended (see chapter 7). It is worth noting that they are used for the management of chronic pain in humans.

Remifentanil is a μ opioid receptor agonist recently introduced for use in humans. It is structurally related to fentanyl and has been developed for use by infusion during anaesthesia. It is an ester which is hydrolysed in plasma and thus is very short-acting. Pharmacokinetic studies in dogs have indicated that the drug is rapidly cleared, the volume of distribution is small and the contribution by the liver to the overall clearance was very low (Chism & Rickert 1996). Therefore this drug has exciting potential for use in dogs during surgery as part of a balanced anaesthetic technique.

Data have been obtained on an oral sustained release preparation of morphine sulphate, as a potentially useful preparation in dogs for the control of moderate to severe pain (Dohoo & Tasker 1997). Absorption of the drug was prolonged (6 h), bioavailability of the drug was low (*c.* 20%) and there was considerable variation between individual dogs. However, the low bioavailability need not restrict the use of this preparation in dogs clinically in the immediate days following major surgery, since low and variable bioavailability is also a characteristic of sustained release morphine preparations in human patients, which are used successfully to manage pain. Clearly, further work should be undertaken to investigate efficacy and safety of this preparation in dogs.

Regulations governing the use of opioid drugs

In the United Kingdom, many of the opioid analgesic drugs are subject to control under the Misuse of Drugs Act 1971, which controls the export, import, production, supply and possession of dangerous drugs. Most other countries have equivalent legislation and this must be observed when using these drugs. In the UK, all the drugs are prescription-only medicines (POMs) and they are allocated into one of five schedules. All the opioid agonists (morphine, diamorphine, etorphine, fentanyl, pethidine, methadone, alfentanil, remifentanil, papaveretum) fall under Schedule 2 and are marked (CD) – Controlled Drug. They must be kept in a locked metal cupboard and records kept of purchases and usage such that on inspection by the Home Office, all drugs can be accounted for. The drugs are subject to special prescription requirements and to legislation on destruction of unwanted stocks. The partial agonists buprenorphine and pentazocine are listed on Schedule 3. Transactions do not have to be recorded in the controlled drugs register for these drugs and prescriptions do not have to be written by hand, but safe-keeping requirements apply to buprenorphine. Schedule 5 includes certain preparations of cocaine, opium, codeine or morphine not hazardous to human health, i.e. they contain less than a specified amount of the drug. They are largely exempt from control, except the need to keep records of purchase for two years. Butorphanol is currently exempt from restriction under the Misuse of Drugs Act. However, since it can induce dependence, although with a low abuse potential, it should be kept under close supervision. Recently butorphanol has become subject to controlled legislation in the USA

There are currently three opioid drugs licensed for use in non-food producing animals: pethidine, butorphanol and buprenorphine; none is licensed for use in food producing animals. In accordance with the Medicines Regulations (1994), which implements parts of the EC Directive 90/676 on veterinary medicine, no veterinary surgeon is allowed to administer a veterinary medicinal product to an animal unless the product has been granted a product licence for the particular species and condition. There are important exceptions to this rule in non-food producing animals such as dogs and cats, and in horses not intended for human consumption. However, legally these drugs cannot be used in food producing animals unless a guarantee can be provided that the animals in question will not enter the food chain.

Non-steroidal antiinflammatory drugs

Pharmacological properties

The non-steroidal antiinflammatory drugs (NSAIDs) are a group of weak organic acids, carboxylic acids (aspirin, cincophen, carprofen, flunixin) and the enolic acids (phenylbutazone, meloxicam), with antiinflammatory, analgesic (peripheral and central sites of action) and antipyretic properties (central site of action). The NSAIDs act by inhibiting the enzymes known as the cyclooxygenases (COX) and thus, they decrease the release of prostaglandins and thromboxane A_2, since COX and lipoxygenases catalyse the conversion of arachidonic acid which is released from cell membranes when they are damaged (Vane 1971). Anti-endotoxaemic effects have been demonstrated for flunixin meglumine at doses considerably less than those required for antiinflammatory or analgesic activity (approx. $\times$ 0.25). Non-steroidal antiinflammatory drugs also have distinct antihyperalgesic properties through a spinal site of action and consequently they play a part in the management of abnormal pain states.

All NSAIDs can have antithrombotic effects by blocking platelet COX (COX-1, see below), and thus inhibiting production of the proaggregatory eicosanoid, thromboxane A_2. However, at therapeutic doses most NSAIDs do not impair clotting mechanisms or prolong bleeding time. Aspirin is unique in this respect since it irreversibly binds to COX so that production of thromboxane A_2 is inhibited for the lifespan of the platelet, and consequently aspirin is a suitable antithrombotic drug.

Two forms of COX have been identified: COX-1, a constitutive enzyme, and COX-2, an inducible enzyme (Xie et al 1991). Until recently, it was considered that the prostaglandins that mediate inflammation, fever and pain were produced by COX-2, while the prostaglandins that are important in gastrointestinal and renal function were produced via COX-1. This led to the belief that the NSAIDs exerted their therapeutically beneficial effects primarily by inhibiting COX-2, while inhibition of COX-1 was considered to be responsible for some of the toxic side-effects associated with these drugs, e.g. gastric ulceration and renal papillary necrosis. Recent work has indicated that the distinction between these two roles is not as clear as was once considered (for review, see Wallace 1999). While highly COX-2 selective drugs (still in development) are gastroprotective and do not induce gastric ulceration, COX-2, while expressed in low amounts in the healthy stomach, appears to play an important role in promoting ulcer healing in the stomach. Consequently, where gastric ulceration is present, COX-2 inhibitors may delay healing. It also appears that COX-1 contributes to the inflammatory process and, consequently, COX-2 selective inhibitors may not be as efficacious as mixed inhibitors in their antiinflammatory actions. COX-2 is consitutively expressed in kidney, and mice which have the COX-2 gene deleted suffer from renal failure and are poorly viable, while displaying inflammatory responses similar to normal mice. Both COX-1 and COX-2 are constitutively expressed in the CNS and their relative expression varies depending on the species. More work is required to elucidate the role of both these enzymes in CNS function. COX-2 generated prostaglandins are also involved in ovulation, parturition and may be involved in wound repair.

Many commercially available NSAIDs at present licensed for use in animals appear to inhibit both enzymes with varying selectivity. There is much controversy over the selectivity of these compounds that are currently licensed, however, with conflicting data being obtained depending on the test systems used for assessing COX-1 and COX-2 selectivity, and also whether these assays are carried out *in vitro, ex vivo* or *in vivo*. In addition, drugs may appear selective for one enzyme over the other while not being highly potent. Currently there are no COX-2 specific drugs licensed for use in veterinary medicine.

Other actions of NSAIDs have been described. An action on prostanoid receptors has been described for meclofenamic acid, while some drugs inhibit β-glucuronidase release from neutrophils. Recent work in humans has indicated a role for COX-2 inhibition in the therapy of colonic cancer. This may represent a new role for NSAID use in the future.

Pharmacokinetics

NSAIDs are generally well absorbed after oral, subcutaneous and intramuscular injection. The presence of food can affect the absorption of some drugs from the gastrointestinal tract in horses (e.g. phenylbutazone). The NSAIDs are all highly protein bound in plasma, more than 99% in some cases, and this can limit the passage of drug from plasma into the interstitial fluid. Most NSAIDs have low volumes of distribution (typically 200–300 ml/kg), although tolfenamic acid has a much greater volume of distribution in dogs. The high degree of protein binding has implications for the use of NSAIDs with other highly protein bound drugs due to saturation of available protein binding sites. Interactions, both therapeutic and toxic, between one NSAID and another are unlikely to be synergistic, but are probably additive. Protein binding explains the extended therapeutic activity in inflamed tissues which many of these drugs display when compared with their plasma elimination half-life. Plasma half-life is, therefore, not the most important factor in determining dosing interval and NSAIDs with even short half-lives such as phenylbutazone (PBZ) and flunixin can be administered once daily to good therapeutic effect (for review, see Lees 1998). Pharmacokinetic data cannot be extrapolated between species, and consequently, dosing schedules must be determined separately for each species.

Metabolism of most NSAIDs occurs in the liver and the metabolites are generally inactive (PBZ is metabolised to the active oxyphenbutazone). If PBZ is given at a high dose level it has a longer half-life in plasma than if it is administered at a lower dose level, i.e. it has dose-dependent kinetics. None of the other NSAIDs licensed for use in animals displays this property. Liver metabolism is important for the inactivation of aspirin, which is conjugated with glucuronic acid. The cat lacks the enzyme glucuronyl transferase and aspirin therefore has a very long half-life in this species, which will lead to drug cumulation and toxicity if the cat is treated like a small dog and dosed accordingly. Aspirin can, however, be used to good therapeutic effect in the cat, although other NSAIDs are now licensed for use in this species (ketoprofen, tolfenamic acid, carprofen). The NSAIDs and their metabolites are mainly excreted via the urine. As they are weak acids, their elimination by the kidney may be influenced by urine pH. Some of the NSAIDs are excreted in the bile as well as via the urine and with these compounds, there may exist a route of enterohepatic recirculation. Currently, there are four NSAIDs licensed for use in food-producing species within the UK: flunixin meglumine, carprofen, ketoprofen and meloxicam.

Toxicity/side-effects

The most commonly encountered toxic side-effect of the NSAIDs is gastrointestinal irritation, which results in ulcer formation and, on occasions, the development of a protein-losing enteropathy. This is a consequence of inhibition of COX-1 which is responsible for the production of prostaglandin PGE_2. This prostaglandin is directly involved in maintaining mucosal blood flow and is also involved in the production of gastric mucus macromolecular glycoproteins which protect the gastric mucosa. NSAIDs may also irritate the stomach mucosa directly (aspirin). Not all NSAIDs have similar ulcerogenic properties. Ulcerogenicity has been determined for many of the NSAIDs; however, there is such a large inter-species variation in metabolism, kinetics and inherent toxicity that it is impossible to extrapolate between species. Recent work in dogs comparing therapeutic doses of meloxicam, carprofen and ketoprofen indicated no significant difference in gastric lesions after seven days therapy (Forsyth et al 1998). Drugs with significant efficacy and potency against COX-1 are highly ulcerogenic. The development of COX-2 selective drugs represents a significant advance in producing antiinflamamatory drugs without gastric side-effects (Cryer 1999). Work in horse intestine *in vitro* has suggested that NSAIDs may have an inhibitory action on smooth muscle. Products which combine an NSAID and misoprostol, a stable derivative of PGE_1, have been developed for use in humans and these products reduce the likelihood of gastric toxicity. Use of misoprostol in dogs significantly inhibits the incidence of flunixin or aspirin induced gastric ulceration (see chapter 6).

Nephrotoxicity is a serious side-effect of these drugs when they are used in animals under conditions of reduced renal blood flow, as occurs frequently during anaesthesia or in hypovolaemic animals (Elwood et al 1992). When renal blood flow falls, PGE_2 (medulla) and PGI_2 (glomerulus) are released into the renal vasculature and cause vasodilatation, thus maintaining renal blood flow. This response is an important component of the kidney's reaction to a fall in arterial blood pressure. If the production of prostaglandins is greatly decreased due the administration of an NSAID, the kidney cannot maintain blood flow. In this situation, nephrotoxicity can result. It is not clear whether this is a COX-1 mediated effect, as work with selective COX-2 inhibitors would suggest that renal side-effects may occur with these drugs. Maintenance of adequate renal perfusion by using minimal amounts of cardiovascular depressant drugs during anaesthesia and attention to fluid therapy reduces the risk of NSAID-induced renal toxicity. The NSAIDs should not be used with other potentially nephrotoxic agents and they should be used with great care in animals with renal disease. Carprofen is an exception to the general rule to avoid using NSAIDs before or during anaesthesia or in animals with compromised renal blood flow, due to its weak inhibition of COX isoenzymes. It has a licence for preoperative use.

Meclofenamic acid has been reported to prolong the gestation period of some species, presumably because of the involvement of prostaglandins in uterine contraction at parturition. It is advisable not to use NSAIDs at this time. They should also be discontinued for five days prior to the use of prostaglandins for breeding purposes.

The effects of NSAIDs on proteoglycan synthesis are not yet fully established. Several NSAIDs, e.g. aspirin, appear to inhibit proteoglycan synthesis; however, results obtained with other NSAIDs depend on whether the cartilage was taken from a weight bearing or non-weight bearing joint, and also on the disease state of the cartilage. Clearly, given the use of these drugs in the management of osteoarthritis in companion animals, a desirable effect would be to stimulate proteoglycan synthesis (Rainsford et al 1999).

Experimental studies with aspirin indicated that the drug was embryotoxic and potentially teratogenic if administered in very early pregnancy; consequently, NSAIDs are contraindicated in pregnant animals. Hepatic toxicity has been associated with phenylbutazone in old horses, and paracetamol is hepatotoxic in many species.

Use of NSAIDs should be avoided in animals receiving concurrent corticosteroid therapy. Corticosteroids inhibit the enzyme phospholipase A_2, an enzyme which liberates arachidonic acid from membrane phospholipid. Since NSAIDs inhibit the enzymes (COX) that catalyse the conversion of arachidonic acid to prostaglandins and thromboxanes, the risk of serious adverse effects if a drug from each class were used in combination would be high. There is a preparation of an NSAID, cinchophen, with a corticosteroid, prednisolone, marketed in the UK for use in dogs with osteoarthritis; however, the relative amount of prednisolone in a given dose is very low.

Individual drugs

The clinical efficacy of the NSAIDs depends upon their pharmacokinetics and upon which cyclooxygenase isoenzymes they are most effective (for review of individual drugs see McKellar et al 1991, Lees 1998). There are many NSAIDs licensed for use in animals and the choice of drug may depend on the individual animal.

Phenylbutazone is still used in the dog and horse in the UK, although this use may be restricted in the future. In the dog, the half-life is short (1–6h) and the active metabolite, oxyphenbutazone, is rapidly eliminated. It has good antiinflammatory activity and is readily administered orally. The strong acidity of the solution makes it too irritant for i.m. or s.c. administration but it can be given by slow i.v. administration, although it may cause thrombophlebitis. Its major use is in the treatment of musculoskeletal inflammatory conditions such as osteoarthritis.

The other enolic NSAID, dipyrone, is used in most domestic species. Dipyrone is combined with hyoscine, a spasmolytic, as 'Buscopan' for use in painful gastrointestinal disorders. Whether it has good effect against visceral pain is not established; however, it is licensed in humans as an analgesic for use in moderate pain. It is rapidly and well absorbed after oral administration.

Cinchophen is an old NSAID which is quite effective in the treatment of osteoarthritis in the dog. It has good analgesic properties but is only weakly antiinflammatory. It has a half-life of 8 h when given with prednisolone. It is only available in combination with the corticosteroid prednisolone (as 'PLT'). Although reportedly quite highly ulcerogenic, studies in dogs indicated that cinchophen–prednisolone combinations produced similar numbers of adverse reactions to therapeutic doses of phenylbutazone.

Flunixin meglumine is an NSAID with very good analgesic, antipyretic and antiinflammatory activity. It is a potent inhibitor of both COX-1 and COX-2 activity. The elimination half-life in most species is short (<6 h), but the duration of effect is considerably longer (12–24 h) due to the cumulation of drug in and slow release of drug from inflamed tissues. It has been used in animals with endotoxic shock. Endotoxin, a lipopolysaccharide produced by gram-negative bacteria, causes eicosanoid production by damaging leukocytes and vascular endothelial cells. The eicosanoids thus generated have a deleterious effect on cardiovascular function. Generation of eicosanoids is inhibited by flunixin and this drug appears to be beneficial in endotoxic shock, even in low doses (0.25 × the antiinflammatory dose), provided it is given early in the course of the syndrome. Flunixin is available as oral and parenteral preparations. Repeat administration of flunixin in cats appears to increase the metabolism of the drug and decrease the duration of action. Flunixin is licensed for use in horses and cattle as an analgesic, antiinflammatory drug and as an antipyretic. It improves the survival and recovery rates of calves with pneumonia when used in combination with antimicrobial therapy. Flunixin toxicity is likely if the dose or dosing interval recommended is exceeded. Gastrointestinal signs and lesions are frequently the first sign of toxicity. Its use peripoperatively should be strictly confined to the *postoperative* period, well into the recovery period, as preoperative administration has been associated with death in dogs from renal failure.

Ketoprofen is licensed for use in the horse, cow, dog and cat and is available in both injection and tablet preparations. It is a potent non-selective inhibitor of COX isoenzymes and is a good antiinflammatory and analgesic agent. It has been used postoperatively to provide analgesia in dogs and cats, and in this respect it has been reported to be effective (Slingsby & Waterman-Pearson 1998). It is a chiral compound and is presented as a racemic mixture. Studies in horses have indicated unidirectional chiral inversion of R(−)– to S(+)–ketoprofen (Landoni & Lees 1996, Landoni et al 1997). Toxicity may limit its use over prolonged periods. Ketoprofen has been used as an antiinflammatory drug in calves with pneumonia and in cows with mastitis.

Tolfenamic acid is licensed for use as an analgesic to treat postoperative pain and to treat acute episodes of chronic musculoskeletal disease and it is licensed for use in cats as an antipyretic and antiinflammatory drug. It is available in both injection and tablet preparations, but its use is restricted to three days. Toxicity may limit its use over prolonged periods.

Carprofen is an NSAID with a single chiral centre which is a poor inhibitor of COX enzymes at therapeutic doses but yet has good antiinflammatory activity. It is presented as a racemic mixture and studies have indicated no chiral inversion of the drug in dogs (McKellar et al 1994). *In vitro* tests suggest that it is COX-2 selective, although not particularly potent in this respect (Ricketts et al 1998). The mode of action is not well understood; however, it is an effective drug in the treatment and management of dogs with degenerative joint disease and in the therapy of acute pain. Studies in dogs undergoing surgery indicated that at the doses recommended, carprofen was as effective as an opioid drug in controlling postoperative pain. The half-life of carprofen varies considerably depending on the species, e.g. approx. 8 h in the dog and approx. 24 h in sheep. It is well absorbed from the GIT and is suitable for once daily administration, although frequently the daily dose is divided in two treatments. Carprofen appears to have a wide safety margin for gastric ulceration, which may reflect its poor activity as a COX inhibitor, and at therapeutic doses it is chondroprotective (*in vitro* studies). A report of hepatocellular toxicosis potentially associated with carprofen administration was recently made (MacPhail et al 1998). This idiosyncratic reaction has not been confirmed in other centres. Carprofen is licensed in the cat for single dose administration; it is effective as a postoperative analgesic and as an inhibitor of experimentally induced inflammation. Carprofen is also licensed in horses for the therapy of pain and in calves for the therapy of acute inflammation associated with respiratory disease.

Meloxicam has been licensed for use in dogs for medium to long term therapy of musculoskeletal pain and inflammation, and is available as a suspension and in injectable form. It is available as an antiinflammatory drug for use in the therapy of calf pneumonia. Meloxicam displays selectivity for the COX-2 isoenzyme in comparison with the COX-1 enzyme. Meloxicam is completely absorbed from the gastrointestinal tract and has a long elimination half-life in the dog (24 h) and is recommended for daily administration. Studies in laboratory animals have indicated that meloxicam does not have a detrimental effect on articular cartilage when used over a prolonged period.

Local anaesthetics

Pharmacological properties

These drugs act to decrease or prevent the large transient increase in the permeability of excitable membranes to Na^+ that normally occurs when the membrane is slightly depolarised (Butterworth & Strichartz 1990). Thus, they stop the transfer of noxious information from the periphery along peripheral nerves. These drugs can provide complete analgesia when applied to tissues. $A\delta$ fibres are most susceptible to blockade followed by C fibres and then by large myelinated fibres. Pain is thus the first sensation to be abolished. The duration of action of a local anaesthetic is dependent on the time that the drug is in contact with the nerve, which is governed by the lipid solubility of the drug, the blood flow to the tissue and the pH of the tissue. To prolong the duration of action, a vasoconstrictor is frequently included in the preparation (usually adrenaline). Vasoconstrictors are normally avoided in solutions used for epidural injection of local anaesthetics.

Amide-linked local anaesthetic drugs (the most commonly used in veterinary practice, lidocaine, mepivacaine, bupivacaine) are bound to $\alpha1$-acid glycoprotein to a varying extent (55–95% in humans). They are degraded in the liver. In humans with severe hepatic disease, these drugs are used with care. Ester-linked local anaesthetics (e.g. procaine) are hydrolysed and inactivated primarily by plasma esterases, probably plasma cholinesterase.

In addition to blocking conduction in peripheral nerve fibres, local anaesthetics in doses higher than those required to induce peripheral blockade have other effects. Paradoxically, in the central nervous system local anaesthetic drugs induce stimulation, restlessness and convulsions, which are ultimately followed by depression. These effects are most commonly observed after inadvertent i.v. administration. Convulsions can be controlled with a benzodiazepine tranquilliser such as diazepam or midazolam. It is essential to provide ventilatory support where respiration is compromised.

Local anaesthetics also act on the myocardium to decrease electrical excitability, conduction rate and force of contraction. Indeed the local anaesthetic drug lidocaine is used acutely to treat cardiac dysrythmias. They may also induce arteriolar dilatation which results in hypotension. Local anaesthetics administered by epidural injection may cause sympathetic blockade and a fall in arterial blood pressure, which can be prevented by administering fluids. The cardiotoxicity of local anaesthetics is most pronounced with bupivacaine given in high doses inadvertently.

Route and method of administration

Local anaesthetic drugs are used topically, e.g. in ear preparations; by local infiltration direct into wound edges; by injection to abolish sensation in a body region, e.g. intercostal nerve blocks; by intrapleural administration; by epidural injection or by intravenous injection into a peripheral vein to provide limb analgesia. In humans, they have been used i.v. in low doses to reduce pain associated with injection of some i.v. anaesthetic agents. However, local anaesthetics have significant side-effects (see below) and should be used with care by the intravenous route.

Use of local anaesthetics

Local anaesthetics are used to provide complete analgesia to allow surgical procedures to be performed in the conscious or sedated animal. They may be used pre-emptively before the onset of tissue damage (e.g. epidural use before hindlimb surgery). They are used to provide analgesia intraoperatively in the anaesthetised animal in order to reduce the amount of general anaesthetic required to obtund responses to painful surgical procedures. They may be employed to control postoperative pain, e.g. intercostal nerve block to reduce pain after thoracotomy.

Individual drugs

Lidocaine is a short-acting drug with a rapid onset of action and a maximum duration of action of approximately 0.75–1 h. This may be extended by incorporating a vasoconstrictor, e.g. adrenaline, in the preparation.

Bupivacaine is a long-acting drug with a slow onset time (peak effect occurs within 30 min). The duration of action varies from 2–6 h, depending on route of administration and the dose. It is used as a 0.25% or 0.5% solution. This drug is not licensed for use in any animal species, although is has been used widely in dogs. It is more cardiotoxic than equieffective doses of lidocaine. Clinically, this is manifested by ventricular arrhythmias and myocardial depression after inadvertent i.v. administration or overdosing in small animals. Generally speaking, the levo stereoisomer of amide local anaesthetics has a lower potential for systemic toxicity than the dextro form of the drug while retaining efficacy, and levobupivacaine is currently under investigation.

Mepivacaine is a local anaesthetic drug that is widely used in equine medicine. It has a duration of action similar to lidocaine.

Ropivacaine, a homologue of mepivacaine and bupivacaine, is a local anaesthetic drug recently licensed for use in humans. It is an enantiomerically pure (S-enantiomer) amide local anaesthetic drug which has greater selectivity for nerve fibres responsible for transmission of pain (Aδ and C fibres) than for those that control motor function (Aβ fibres) in *in vitro* studies, although this is dose dependent (Markham & Faulds 1996). Its clinical efficacy appears to be quite similar to that of bupivacaine but it has a greater margin of safety. Ropivacaine is less cardiotoxic than bupivacaine. It has a similar onset time and duration of action. Epidural ropivacaine is less potent than epidural bupivacaine when the two drugs are administered at the same concentration, although this difference is less marked in terms of sensory blockade than motor blockade.

The use of topical local anaesthesia is employed on occasions, although more commonly for diagnostic or surgical purposes. A eutectic mixture of local anaesthetics, EMLA has been developed for topical application to achieve cutaneous anaesthesia. EMLA cream contains the amide local anaesthetics lidocaine and prilocaine, and is applied to the area of skin to be anaesthetised; it is covered by a dressing for a minimum of 60 minutes. In humans, the duration of analgesia lasts for several hours. When applied to diseased skin, the duration of action is shorter as the local anaesthetics are absorbed more quickly. It has been used with good success in fractious animals, to facilitate venepuncture.

Alpha-2 adrenoceptor agonists

These drugs – xylazine, medetomidine, detomidine and romifidine – produce analgesia by binding to alpha$_2$ receptors present in the CNS. Alpha-2 adrenoceptors, which exist as four different subtypes, are located in structures closely related to pain information processing within the brain and spinal cord and in other tissues throughout the body. They are generally inhibitory in function on cells. Their primary use in veterinary medicine is in producing sedation, while they are commonly used in humans to manage hypertension. They are potent analgesics in most species (Nolan et al 1987); however, their usefulness in this respect is restricted by dose-dependent sedation and cardiovascular depression (Khan et al 1999).

Alpha-2 adrenoceptor agonists induce dose-dependent sedation in all domestic animals, although their efficacy in pigs is less than in other species. They induce dose-related cardiovascular depression which varies according to the drug used. Cardiac output is reduced and bradycardia is present, which can be marked. Vomiting is frequently observed in the dog and cat; the incidence appears to be related to the particular drug used. Gut motility is inhibited in all species as alpha-2 adrenoceptors are located presynaptically on parasympathetic nerve terminals in intestinal smooth muscle. Here, they inhibit the release of acetylcholine onto intestinal muscarinic receptors and hence decrease gut motility. They induce variable degrees of respiratory depression. In sheep, these drugs can induce dyspnoea and severe arterial hypoxaemia and they are best avoided in this species or used only with extreme care (Waterman et al 1987). They induce hormonal and metabolic alterations, e.g. antidiuretic hormone production is decreased and growth hormone release is increased. They are administered parenterally, either i.m., s.c. or i.v.

At the dose rates recommended in the data sheets, these drugs are not commended for use as analgesics, as the cardiovascular depression is considered too great. They are commonly used in horses to control pain associated with colic (Nolan 1995), for which purpose their sedative properties are particularly useful. Related drugs, clonidine and dexmedetomidine, have been used epidurally and intrathecally in humans as part of an analgesic regime for the management of severe pain, both acute and chronic, and as a part of a balanced anaesthetic technique. They are frequently combined with opioids or local anaesthetics drugs when given by this route. Xylazine has been used epidurally in cattle, horses and sheep with good success, although the effects are not long lasting. Use of medetomidine by the epidural route in cows is associated with long-lasting analgesia. Alpha-2 adrenoceptor agonists may be useful analgesics in other species when used at low doses, alone or in combination with opioids (see chapter 5). Xylazine is licensed for use in cattle in the UK and consequently can be used in other animals intended for human consumption provided the standard meat and milk withdrawal times are observed. Atipamezole is an alpha-2 antagonist which will antagonise the effects of agonist drugs of this class.

Miscellaneous drugs

Ketamine

Ketamine is a non-competitive antagonist of the N-methyl-D-asparate (NMDA) receptor, one of the excitatory amino acid receptors at which glutamate acts (see chapter 2). This receptor is intimately involved in the induction and maintenance of altered pain responses following trauma/inflammation (chapter 2). Therefore, antagonists of the receptor appear to have some analgesic and antihyperalgesic properties. Ketamine is presented as a mixture of isomers and there is some evidence to suggest that the R(−) isomer is associated with excitatory effects while the S(+) isomer is associated with pain modulating effects. S(+) ketamine is currently being evaluated in humans for use as an adjunct to total intravenous anaesthesia. The use of ketamine is restricted due to excitatory actions within the CNS. Ketamine is one of very few drugs used perioperatively to have stimulatory effects on the cardiovascular system. These are mediated through the sympathetic nervous system. Ketamine can cause respiratory depression. It is primarily used as an anaesthetic agent in horses, cats and rabbits, following premedication with an alpha-2 adrenoceptor agonist drug. Dogs appear to be particularly sensitive to the excitatory effects of ketamime. Work in humans has indicated that ketamine may be effective in reversing some chronic pain states, e.g. phantom limb pain, and it is used for particularly painful procedures, e.g. changing burn dressings. Ketamine may have a role as an analgesic at low doses in cats and it has been used with good success to suppress responses to surgical stimulation in horses during anaesthesia, and by intravenous infusion in horses (Nolan et al 1997) and perioperatively in dogs (Lerche et al 2000).

Nitrous oxide

Nitrous oxide, a gas delivered to the patient by inhalation, is a good analgesic in humans, and it is used routinely to provide analgesia during surgery and anaesthesia. It has low potency in domestic animals; however, when administered at a concentration of ?60–70% it appears to have some analgesic properties. It is used as an adjunct to inhalational or intravenous anaesthesia; it does not provide lasting analgesia and once administration of nitrous oxide is discontinued the effects wane rapidly (within 5 min).

Future targets for analgesic drug development

Many neurotransmitters and their receptors have been implicated in the induction and maintenance of inflammatory and neuropathic pain and hyperalgesia and allodynia, and over the next decade it is anticipated that new analgesic drugs and therapies will appear for the relief and management of pain in humans and animals. The excitatory peptide neurotransmitter, substance P, acting at the neurokinin 1 receptor, is intimately involved in the induction of 'wind-up' in the spinal cord (see chapter 5). Neurokinin 1 receptor antagonists have proved useful in experimental models of pain although their use in clinical trials in humans has been disappointing. The identification of tetrodotoxin-resistant sodium channels in peripheral sensory nerves opens the possibility of developing channel blockers (local anaesthetics) which do not affect motor nerve function. Vanilloid receptors which are involved in mediating specific types of pain may be suitable for manipulation, and antagonists of these receptors may be analgesic. Nicotinic agonists of a particular subunit structure (e.g. epibatidine) have been reported to be potent effective analgesics in laboratory animal species, although curently side-effects restrict their use. A role for metabotropic glutamate receptors in modifying nociception has been established and once selective antagonists are developed, further information on this complex receptor system will become available. δ opioid agonists are under rigorous study and development, as they produce analgesia without the side-effects of respiratory depression or habituation. Modulation of the γ-aminobutyric acid (GABA) A receptor/benzodiazepine complex has been effective in some pain states. Further study in this field is underway. The antiepileptic drug, gabapentin, has potent analgesic and antihyperalgesic properties in both inflammatory and neuropathic pain, although its antinociceptive mode of action is unclear. Nerve growth factor is ultimately involved in spinal cord reorganization following noxious stimuli and modulation of this neurotrophin may prove clinically effective in the future. Gene therapy efforts aimed at managing chronic pain have been initiated and successful transfer of genes to the meninges surrounding the spinal cord has been achieved *in vivo*.

These are but some of the many avenues of research currently under investigation and in time it is likely that new therapies for pain will emerge to promote the ability of physicians and veterinary surgeons to manage pain more effectively in the future.

Corticosteroids

Corticosteroids are not analgesic drugs; however, as potent antiinflammatory agents, they may have a role to play in treating medically painful inflammatory conditions, e.g. otitis externa, osteoarthritis. Their pharmacology will be described briefly (for review, see Nolan 1998).

Glucocorticoids exert their effects on cellular metabolism through the interaction with specific hormone receptors located intracellularly. They induce the transcription of specific mRNAs which result in new protein synthesis; they also switch off the production of some proteins. They inhibit the induction of COX-2 and inducible nitric oxide synthase. One of the proteins induced is lipocortin (more correctly, a family of proteins), which appears to be a specific inhibitor of phospholipase A_2. Inhibition of phospholipase A_2, which catalyses the release of arachidonic acid from cell membranes, prevents the release of prostaglandins, thromboxane and leukotrienes which are important mediators of both the early and late responses to inflammation. Inhibition of phospholipase A_2 is not the sole mechanism by which glucocorticoids induce their antiinflammatory effect: the corticosteroids are also thought to stabilise and maintain the integrity of cellular, lysosomal and mitochondrial membranes.

Corticosteroids are well absorbed if given orally and are generally administered by this route to animals on medium or long-term therapy. Parenteral therapy is generally used to initiate a course of short-term therapy, although depot preparations with long duration of action are available. Glucocorticoids are metabolised primarily in the liver, where they are reduced and conjugated with glucuronic acid, and are then excreted in the urine. Glucocorticoids may be formulated in a number of ways which will confer therapeutically desirable characteristics, e.g. for topical application, acetonide esters are particularly useful.

The most important clinical effect of glucocorticoid therapy is on inflammation and the antiinflammatory effects are complex. Corticosteroids suppress both the early and later stages of inflammation. Other effects include increased gluconeogenesis and inhibition of peripheral utilisation of glucose, catabolic effects on proteins, and redistribution of body fat. Reduction in cellular migration to inflammatory sites, osteoporosis, induction of hepatic enzymes and potential retention of Na^+ and H_2O and excretion of H^+ and K^+ are other effects.

Toxicity to corticosteroids is common. Two main syndromes occur: that associated with long-term high-dosage administration is iatrogenic Cushing's syndrome. The risk of inducing Cushing's syndrome is reduced by administering minimal doses of steroid for long-term therapy and instituting alternative day therapy wherever possible with short-acting glucocorticoids such as prednisolone.

Excessive use of glucocorticoids also induces adrenal hypofunction and atrophy as a consequence of suppression of the hypothalamic-pituitary-adrenal (HPA) axis by negative feedback. Abrupt termination of prolonged therapy leaves the animal with a poorly functioning adrenal cortex which is unable to respond to stress and may lead to an Addisonian type crisis. In order to avoid adrenal atrophy, an alternate day regime has been developed for corticosteroid administration which depends on the administration of a high dose level of a short-acting corticosteroid every alternate day. This regimen allows the adrenal gland to recover on the following day, during which there is no exogenous steroid administration, and thus no negative feedback on the gland. This system of alternate day therapy has been shown to produce significantly less adrenal suppression in dogs.

Actions upon the gut may lead to gastric ulceration and, in extreme cases, perforation. Glucocorticoids may potentiate the ulcerogenic effects of non-steroidal antiinflammatory drugs and concurrent therapy should be avoided. Dogs undergoing spinal surgery which are treated with corticosteroids are particularly susceptible to intestinal ulceration (stomach or colon) severe enough to cause perforation. Thus in dogs undergoing spinal surgery that receive treatment with corticosteroids, adjunct therapy with a histamine antagonist such as ranitidine is recommended. Muscle atrophy, and cutaneous atrophy with calcium deposition in the skin, are other side-effects of long-term corticosteroid therapy. The hyperglycaemia associated with glucocorticoids precludes their use in animals with diabetes mellitus and indeed this condition may be unmasked by glucocorticoid activity. The osteoporotic effect due to decreased calcium absorption and increased renal excretion limits their use in rapidly growing dogs, particularly of the larger breeds. All the corticosteroids have some mineralocorticoid effect, which causes sodium and water retention and which may induce oedema. Consequently, they are best avoided in patients with congestive heart failure. They also cause hypokalaemia and alkalosis because of increased loss of potassium and hydrogen ions.

Principles of therapy

It is imperative to remember that treatment with the corticosteroids is purely palliative except where there is a primary adrenal cortical insufficiency. The more potent and long-acting compounds are associated with greater risk of toxicity.

Clinical use

Corticosteroids are indicated in acute conditions where the inflammatory response is more damaging than the underlying condition, e.g. iritis, uveitis, where the animal may inflict further trauma upon itself by rubbing, etc. In all inflammatory conditions they should be used in combination with appropriate therapy for the underlying cause and corticosteroids should be withdrawn gradually from the therapeutic regime as early as possible.

Corticosteroids have been used for the treatment of osteoarthritic conditions and in some cases are considered to be useful, e.g. in animals that are unable to tolerate non-steroidal antiinflammatory drugs or where there is a significant inflammatory component to the disease. However, since they have osteoporotic side-effects, although these effects are not commonly observed in dogs, long-term therapy is ill-advised. At low doses, corticosteroids may be useful in the early stages of degenerative joint disease in delaying the osteophyte production and inhibiting degradative enzyme production.

References

Atweh, S.F. and Kuhar, M.J. (1977a) Autoradiographic localization of opiate receptors in rat brain. I. Spinal cord and lower medulla. Brain Research **124**: 53–67.

Atweh, S.F. and Kuhar, M.J. (1977b) Autoradiographic localization of opiate receptors in rat brain. II. The brain stem. Brain Research **129**: 1–12.

Atweh, S.F. and Kuhar, M.J. (1977c) Autoradiographic localization of opiate receptors in rat brain. III. The telencephalon. Brain Research **134**: 393–405.

Barnhart, M.D., Hubbell, J.A.E., Muir, W.W., et al (2000) Pharmacokinetics, pharmacodynamics, and analgesic effects of morphine. American Journal of Veterinary Research **61**: 24–28.

Benthuysen, J. L. and Stanley, T. H. (1985) Concerning the possible nature of reported fentanyl seizures. Anesthesiology **62**: 205–209.

Bolser, D.C. (1996) Mechanisms of action of central and peripheral antitussive drugs. Pulmonary Pharmacology and Therapeutics **9**: 357–364.

Butterworth, J.F. and Strichartz, G.R. (1990) Molecular mechanisms of local anesthesia: a review. Anesthesiology **72**: 711–734.

Chism, J.P. and Rickert, D.E. (1996) The pharmacokinetics and extra-hepatic clearance of remifentanil in male beagle dogs during constant rate infusions. Drug Metabolism and Disposition **24**: 34–40.

Combie, J., Dougherty, J., Nugent, E. and Tobin, T. (1981) Pharmacology of narcotic analgesics in the horse. American Journal of Veterinary Research **42**: 716–721.

Concannon, K.T., Dodam, J.R. and Hellyer, P.W. (1995) Influence of a mu- and kappa-opioid agonist on isoflurane minimal anesthetic concentration in chickens. American Journal of Veterinary Research **56**: 806–811.

Court, M.H., Dodman, N.H., Levine, H.D., et al (1992) Pharmacokinetics and milk residues of butorphanol in dairy cows after single intravenous administration. Journal of Veterinary Pharmacology and Therapeutics **15**: 28–35.

Cryer, B. (1999) Current Opinion in Gastroenterology 15: 473–480.

Dohoo, S.E. and Tasker, R.A.R. (1997) Pharmacokinetics of oral morphine sulfate in dogs. Canadian Journal of Veterinary Research **61**: 251–255.

Elwood, C., Boswood, A., Simpson, K. and Carmichael, S. (1992) Renal failure after flunixin meglumine administration. Veterinary Record **130**: 582–583.

Florez, J., McCarthy, L.E. and Borison, H.L. (1968) A comparative study in the cat of the respiratory effects of morphine injected intravenously and into the cerebrospinal fluid. Journal of Pharmacology and Experimental Therapeutics **163**: 448–455.

Forsyth, S.F., Guilford, W.G., Haslett, S.J. and Godfrey, J. (1998) Endoscopy of the gastroduodenal mucosa after carprofen, meloxicam and ketoprofen administration in dogs. Journal of Small Animal Practice **39**: 421–424.

Fox, S.M., Mellor, D.J., Lawoko, C.R.O., et al (1998) Changes in plasma cortisol concentrations in bitches in response to different combinations of halothane and butorphanol. Research in Veterinary Science **65**: 125–133.

Freye, E. (1974) Cardiovascular effects of high dosages of fentanyl, meperidine, and naloxone in dogs. Anesthesia and Analgesia **53**: 40–47.

Fukuda, K., Kato, S., Mori, K., et al (1994) cDNA cloning and regional distribution of a novel member of the opioid receptor family. FEBS Letters **343**: 42–46.

Garner, H.R., Burke, T.F., Lawhorn, C.D., et al (1997) Butorphanol-mediated antinociception in mice: partial agonist effects and mu receptor involvement. Journal of Pharmacology and Experimental Therapeutics **282**: 1253–1261.

Garrett, E.R. and Chandran, V.R. (1990) Pharmacokinetics of morphine and its surrogates. Biopharmaceutics and Drug Disposition **11**: 311–350.

Goldstein, A., Lowney, L.I. and Pal, M. (1971) Stereospecific and nonspecific interactions of the morphine congener levorphanol in subcellular fractions of mouse brain. Proceedings of the National Academy of Sciences USA **68**: 1742–1747.

Heine, M.F., Tillet, E.D., Tsueda, K., et al (1994) Intra-articular morphine after arthroscopic knee operation. British Journal of Anaesthesia **73**: 413–415.

Hoke, J.F., Cunningham, F., James, M.K., et al (1997) Comparative pharmacokinetics and pharmacodynamics of remifentanil, its principle metabolite (GR90291) and alfentanil in dogs. Journal of Pharmacology and Experimental Therapeutics **281**: 226–232.

Horan, P. and Ho, I.K. (1991) The physical dependence liability of butorphanol: a comparative study with morphine. European Journal of Pharmacology **203**: 387–391.

49

Hustveit, O. and Setekleiv, J. (1993) Fentanyl and pethidine are antagonists on muscarinic receptors in guinea-pig ileum. Acta Anaesthesiologica Scandinavica **37**: 541–544.

Ilkiw, J.E., Pascoe, P.J. and Fisher, L.D. (1997) Effect of alfentanil on the minimum alveolar concentration of isoflurane in cats. American Journal of Veterinary Research **58**: 1274–1279.

Jacqz, E., Ward, S., Johnson, R., et al (1986) Extrahepatic glucuronidation of morphine in the dog. Drug Metabolism and Disposition **14**: 627–630.

Johnson, C.B. and Taylor, P.M. (1997) Effects of alfentanil on the equine electroencephalogram during anaesthesia with halothane in oxygen. Research in Veterinary Science **62**: 159–163.

Joshi, G.P., McSwiney, M., Hurson, B.J., et al (1993) Effects of intraarticular morphine on analgesic requirements after anterior cruciate ligament repair. Regional Anesthesia **18**: 254–257.

Kapas, S., Purbrick, A. and Hinson, J.P. (1995) Action of opioid peptides on the rat adrenal cortex: stimulation of steroid secretion through a specific mu opioid receptor. Journal of Endocrinology **144**: 503–510.

Khan, Z.P., Ferguson, C.N. and Jones, R.M. (1999) Alpha-2 and imidazoline receptor agonists. Their pharmacology and therapeutic role. Anaesthesia **54**: 146–165.

Kromer, W. (1988) Endogenous and exogenous opioids in the control of gastrointestinal motility and secretion. Pharmacological Reviews **40**: 121–162.

Kyles, A.E. (1998) Transdermal fentanyl. Compendium on Continuing Education for the Practicing Veterinarian **20**: 721–726.

Kyles, A.E., Papich, M. and Hardie, E.M. (1996) Disposition of transdermally administered fentanyl in dogs. American Journal of Veterinary Research **57**: 715–719.

Landoni, M.F. and Lees, P. (1996) Pharmacokinetics and pharmacodynamics of ketoprofen enantiomers in the horse. Journal of Veterinary Pharmacology and Therapeutics **19**: 466–474.

Landoni, F., Soraci, A.L., Delatour, P. and Lees, P. (1997) Enantioselective behaviour of drugs used in domestic animals: a review. Journal of Veterinary Pharmacology and Therapeutics **20**: 1–16.

Lees, P. (1998) Non-steroidal anti-inflammatory drugs. In: Canine Medicine and Therapeutics. Gorman, N.T. (ed) pp 106–118.

Lees, P. and Hillidge, C.J. (1975) Influence of the neuroleptanalgesic combination of etorphine and acepromazine on the horse. Equine Veterinary Journal **7**: 184–191.

Lees, P. and Hillidge, C.J. (1976) Immobilon: comments on its action. Veterinary Record **99**: 55–56.

Lerche, P., Nolan, A.M. and Reid, J. (2000) propofol or propofol and ketamine for induction of anaesthesia in the dog: a comparative study. Veterinary Record (in press).

McKellar, Q.A., Delatour, P. and Lees, P. (1994) Stereospecific pharmacodynamics and pharmacokinetics of carprofen in the dog. Journal of Veterinary Pharmacology and Therapeutics **17**: 447–454.

McKellar, Q.A., May, S.A. and Lees, P. (1991) Journal of Small Animal Practice **32**: 225–235.

MacPhail, C.M., Lappin, M.R., Meyer, D.J., et al (1998) Hepatocellular toxicosis associated with administration of carprofen in 21 dogs. Journal of the American Veterinary Medical Association **212**: 1895–1901.

Markham, A. and Faulds, D. (1996) Ropivacaine. A review of its pharmacology and therapeutic use in regional anaesthesia. Drugs **52**: 429–449.

Matthews, N.S. and Lindsay, S.L. (1990) Effect of low-dose butorphanol on halothane minimum alveolar concentration in ponies. Equine Veterinary Journal **22**: 325–327.

Martin, W.R. (1984) Pharmacology of opioids. Pharmacological Reviews **35**: 283–323.

Meunier, J.C., Mollereau, C., Toll, L., et al (1995) Isolation and structure of the endogenous agonist of opioid receptor-like ORL1 receptor. Nature **377**: 532–535.

Merrell, W.J., Gordon, L., Wood, A.J.J., et al (1990) The effect of halothane on morphine disposition. Anesthesiology **72**: 308–314.

Michelsen, L.G., Salmenpera, M., Hug, C.C., et al (1996) Anesthetic potency of remifentanil in dogs. Anesthesiology **84**: 865–872.

Minami, M. and Satoh, M. (1995) Molecular biology of the opioid receptors: structures, functions and distributions. Neuroscience Research **23**: 121–145.

Moore, A.S., Rand, W.M., Berg, J., et al (1994) Evaluation of butorphanol and cyproheptadine for prevention of cisplatin-induced vomiting in dogs. Journal of the American Veterinary Medical Association **205**: 441–443.

Nolan, A. (1995) In: The Equine Manual. Higgins, A.J. and Wright, I.M. (eds).

Nolan, A. (1998) In: Canine Medicine and Therapeutics. Ed. Gorman, N.T. pp 94–105.

Nolan, AM. and Hall, LW. (1984) Combined use of sedatives and opiates in horses. Veterinary Record **114**: 63–67.

Nolan, A.M., Chambers, J.P. and Hale, G.J. (1991) The cardiorespiratory effects of morphine and butorphanol in horses anaesthetised under clinical conditions. Journal of Veterinary Anaesthesia **18**: 19–24.

Nolan, A., Livingston, A. and Waterman, A. (1987) Antinociceptive actions of intravenous alpha 2-adrenoceptor agonists in sheep. Journal of Veterinary Pharmacology and Therapeutics **10**: 202–209.

Nolan, A.M. and Reid, J. (1991) The use of intraoperative fentanyl in spontaneously breathing dogs undergoing orthopaedic surgery. Journal of Veterinary Anaesthesia **18**: 30–34.

Nolan, A.M., Besley, W., Reid, J. and Gray, G. (1994) The effects of butorphanol on locomotor activity in ponies: a preliminary study. Journal of Veterinary Pharmacology and Therapeutics **17**: 323–326.

Nolan, A., Waterman, A.E. and Livingston, A. (1988) The correlation of the thermal and mechanical antinociceptive activity of pethidine hydrochloride with plasma concentrations of the drug in sheep. Journal of Veterinary Pharmacology and Therapeutics **11**: 94–102.

Pascoe, P.J. (1992) Advantages and guidelines for using epidural drugs for analgesia. Veterinary Clinics of North America Small Animal Practice **22**: 421–423.

Pascoe, P.J., Black, W.D., Claxton, J.M., and Sansom, R.E. (1991) The pharmacokinetics and locomotor activity of alfentanil in the horse. Journal of Veterinary Pharmacology and Therapeutics **14**: 317–325.

Pascoe, P.J., Steffey, E.P., Black, W.D., et al (1993) Evaluation of the effect of alfentanil on the minimum alveolar concentration of halothane in horses. American Journal of Veterinary Research **54**: 1327–1332.

Peacock, J.E. and Francis, G. (1997) Drugs of Today **33**: 611–618.

Pert, C. and Snyder, S. (1973) Opiate receptor. Science **179**: 1011–1014.

Pfeffer, M., Smyth, R.D., Pittman, K.A. and Nardella, P.A. (1980) Pharmacokinetics of subcutaneous and intramuscular butorphanol in dogs. Journal of Pharmaceutical Sciences **69**: 801–803.

Pfeiffer, A. (1990) In: Neurobiology of Opioids. Almeida, O. and Shippenberg, T. (eds). Springer-Verlag, pp 351–362.

Rainsford, K.D., Skerry, T.M., Chindemi, P. and Delaney, K. (1999) Effects of the NSAIDs meloxicam and indomethacin on cartilage proteoglycan synthesis and joint responses to calcium pyrophosphate crystals in dogs. Veterinary Research Communications **23**: 101–113.

Ricketts, A.P., Lundy, K.M. and Seibel, S.B. (1998) Evaluation of selective inhibition of canine cyclooxygenase 1 and 2 by carprofen and other nonsteroidal anti-inflammatory drugs. American Journal of Veterinary Research **59**: 1441–1446.

Sawyer, D.C., Rech, R.H., Durham, R.A., et al (1991) Dose response to butorphanol administered subcutaneously to increase visceral nociceptive threshold in dogs. American Journal of Veterinary Research **52**: 1826–1830.

Schlarmann, B., Gorlitz, B.D., Wintzer, H.J. and Frey, H.H. (1973) Clinical pharmacology of an etorphine-acepromazine preparation. American Journal of Veterinary Research **34**: 411–415.

Scherk-Nixon, M (1996) A study of the use of a transdermal fentanyl patch in cats. Journal of the American Animal Hospital Association **32**: 19–24.

Simonin, F., Valverde, O., Smadja, C., et al (1998) Disruption of the kappa–opioid receptor gene in mice enhances sensitivity to chemical visceral pain, impairs pharmacological actions of the selective kappa-agonist U-50,488H and attenuates morphine withdrawal. EMBO Journal **17**: 886–897.

Slingsby, L.S. and Waterman-Pearson, A.E. (1998) Comparison of pethidine, buprenorphine and ketoprofen for postoperative analgesia after ovariohysterectomy in the cat. Veterinary Record **143**: 185–189.

Stein, C. (1993) Peripheral mechanisms of opioid analgesia. Anesthesia and Analgesia **6**: 182–191.

Steffey, E.P., Baggot, J.D., Eisele, J.H., et al (1994) Morphine-isoflurane interaction in dogs, swine and rhesus monkeys. Journal of Veterinary Pharmacology and Therapeutics **17**: 202–210.

Valverde, A., Dyson, D.H. and McDonell, W.N. (1989) Epidural morphine reduces halothane MAC in the dog. Canadian Journal of Anaesthesia **36**: 629–632.

Van Ham, L.M.L., Nijs, J., Mattheeuws, D.R.G., and Vanderstraeten, G.G.W. (1996) Sufentanil and nitrous oxide anaesthesia for the recording of transcranial magnetic motor evoked potentials in dogs. Veterinary Record **138**: 642–645.

Vane, J. R. (1971) Inhibition of prostaglandin synthesis as a mechanism of action for aspirin-like drugs. Nature **231**: 232–235.

Walker, D.J. and Zacny, J.P. (1999) Subjective, psychomotor, and physiological effects of cumulative doses of opioid mu agonists in healthy volunteers. Journal of Pharmacology and Experimental Therapeutics **289**: 1454–1464.

Wallace, J.L. (1999) Selective COX-2 inhibitors. Trends in Pharmacological Sciences, **20**: 4–6.

Waterman, A.E., Livingston, A. and Amin, A. (1990) The antinociceptive activity and respiratory effects of fentanyl in sheep. Journal of the Association of Veterinary Anaesthetists **17**: 20–23.

Waterman, A.E. and Kalthum, W. (1989) Pharmacokinetics of intramuscularly administered pethidine in dogs and the influence of anaesthesia and surgery. Veterinary Record **124**: 293–296.

Waterman, A.E. and Kalthum, W. (1990) Pharmacokinetics of pethidine administered intramuscularly and intravenously to dogs over 10 years old. Research in Veterinary Science **48**: 245–248.

Waterman, A.E., Nolan, A.M. and Livingston, A. (1987) Influence of idazoxan on the respiratory blood gas changes induced by alpha 2-adrenoceptor agonist drugs in conscious sheep. Veterinary Record **121**: 105–107.

Wamsley, J.K., Zarbin, M.A., Young, W.S. and Kuhar, M.J. (1982) Distribution of opiate receptors in the monkey brain: an autoradiographic study. Neuroscience **7**: 595–613.

Willens, J.S. and Myslinski, N.R. (1993) Pharmacodynamics, pharmacokinetics, and clinical uses of fentanyl, sufentanil, and alfentanil. Heart and Lung **22**: 239–251.

Xie, W., Chipman, J.G., Robertson, D.L., et al (1991) Expression of a mitogen-responsive gene encoding prostaglandin synthase is regulated by mRNA splicing. Proceedings of the National Academy of Sciences USA **88**: 1692–1696.

Zaki, P.A., Bilsky, E.J., Vanderah, T.W., et al (1996) Opioid receptor types and subtypes. Annual Review of Pharmacology and Toxicology **36**: 379–401.

PAIN ASSESSMENT

4

P. Dobromylskyj, P.A. Flecknell, B.D. Lascelles,
A. Livingston, P. Taylor, A. Waterman-Pearson

Effective pain management can only be achieved and maintained when the signs of pain can be assessed accurately and reliably. The experience of pain is unique to each individual and this perception is translated into and described by verbal descriptions in man. This makes the assessment of pain in animals particularly difficult as there is no verbal means of communication between animals and humans.

This difficulty in assessing pain in animals often results in:

- Analgesics being withheld because the animal shows no overt signs of pain (in other words, it does not behave in a similar way to a human who is experiencing pain)
- An assumption that, since a human who has undergone a similar procedure would require analgesics, the animal must require pain relief, and analgesics are therefore administered.

In the first scenario, animals which are almost certainly in pain will not receive adequate analgesia; in the second case, since no proper assessment of the degree of pain has been made, it is a matter of chance whether an appropriate degree of pain relief is provided. Nevertheless, it is important to emphasise that, in our experience, adopting the latter approach and administering an initial dose of analgesic is almost invariably beneficial, and rarely causes significant clinical side-effects (Flecknell 1994, Lascelles 1996). Administering repeated doses of analgesics to animals which are not experiencing pain may, however, be detrimental – for example, the drug may depress appetite and so delay recovery (Liles & Flecknell 1992a). It is clearly preferable to try to assess the animal's pain, and adjust the analgesic regimen according to the results of this assessment.

Assessment of acute pain responses – analgesiometry

In addition to attempting to assess the severity of pain in clinical situations, the responses to a sudden, acute painful stimulus have been used to determine the efficacy of different analgesics. Since a number of analgesics are also sedative agents, it is often necessary to assess both analgesia and sedation. Most of these investigations have been carried out in rodents, and use mechanical, thermal or electrical stimuli to produce a brief painful stimulus. The majority of studies are designed in such a way that the animal can terminate the stimulus. The various techniques used in rodents have been reviewed (Flecknell 1984, Liles & Flecknell 1992b), and these systems have been modified for use in larger species. For example, Kamerling (Kamerling et al 1989) has undertaken a number of studies investigating analgesics in horses using electrical tooth or hoof stimulation. NSAIDs have been studied using heat applied to the saddle area (Schatzmann et al 1990). Lowe & Hilfiger (1986) investigated visceral analgesia by using balloons inflated in the caecum. In all of these studies analgesic effect was measured by the increase in intensity of the stimulus (pressure, electrical current, etc.) which could be applied before the horses exhibited specified behavioural signs of pain. Thermal and mechanical stimuli have been used in sheep (Nolan et al 1987, 1988) and a colonic balloon model to assess visceral pain has been used in the cat and dog (Sawyer & Rech 1987, Sawyer at al 1991, 1992).

These assessment methods enable a determination of the analgesic potency of different drugs, but the dose rates required vary depending upon the test and the analgesic used. NSAIDs are generally relatively ineffective, and the test systems used require some modification when assessing this class of analgesics. This relative lack of efficacy in response to acute brief noxious stimuli, in comparison with opioids, is sometimes misinterpreted as showing that NSAIDs are therefore unlikely to be effective in controlling clinical pain. This is clearly not the case. It is also difficult to relate the dose rates which are effective in these test systems with those which are needed to control clinical pain. In some instances this can lead to relatively high dose rates of analgesics being recommended for clinical use, but these are usually revised once clinical studies have been carried out.

Assessment of clinical pain

Numerous different methods of assessing pain have been developed in man, and attempts have been made to apply some of these to animals. The use of objective measures, such as heart rate, respiratory rate and temperature are an unreliable guide to the presence of pain (Conzemius et al 1997), as are clinicopathological measurements of humoral factors such as epinephrine (adrenaline), norepinephrine (noradrenaline) and cortisol. These measures may be useful when integrated into a pain scoring system, but since they may be influenced by so many factors other than pain, they are of limited use as predictors of pain severity when used alone. Adult humans have the ability to provide direct verbal communication, to complete pain questionnaires or scoring systems and to manage analgesic dosage directly using patient-controlled analgesia systems. This allows reasonably reliable estimates to be made of the degree of pain and the efficacy of pain control. In young human infants, written and verbal communication is not possible, nevertheless extrapolation from adult humans, coupled with objective demonstrations of the adverse effects of surgical stress, has led to a huge increase in interest in providing pain relief to these patients (Anand et al 1987, McGrath & Unruh 1989, Anand 1990, McGrath 1990).

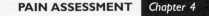

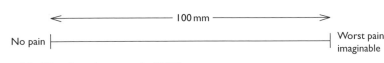

Figure 4.1 Visual analogue scale (VAS).

The approaches used in human infants can provide a framework for animal pain assessment. The most widely used techniques have been pain scoring systems based upon criteria such as crying, facial expression, posture and behaviour (McGrath & Unruh 1989), with these criteria being scored by an experienced observer. The pain scales used have been either simple descriptive scales, numerical rating scales, visual analogue scales or multifactorial pain scales. These have all been adapted for veterinary use, and they are described in more detail below.

The visual analogue scale (VAS) consists of a 100 mm line, anchored at one end 'no pain' and at the other 'excruciating or unbearable pain', or some similar wording (Murrin & Rosen 1985) (Fig. 4.1). The clinician assessing the animal places a mark on the line to indicate the amount of pain they believe the animal to be suffering. The distance from the 'no pain' end of the line (in mm) is the pain score. The numerical rating scale (NRS) is similar, but the observer assigns a numerical score for pain intensity rather than placing a mark on a line. Typically, a scale of 0 to 10 is used. The simple descriptive scale (SDS) consists of four or five expressions used to describe various levels of pain intensity (no pain, mild pain, moderate pain or severe pain). Each expression is assigned an index value, which becomes the pain score for the animal. The mulitifactorial pain scale (MFPS) is usually a composite of a number of SDS values relating to particular aspects of behaviour that may be associated with pain.

The performance of these scales for the assessment of pain in both humans and animals has been investigated. It has been found that the SDS is less sensitive than the VAS or the NRS (Scott and Huskissen 1976). Good agreement has been found between the VAS and an NRS system when assessing lameness in sheep, but with the VAS being more sensitive (Welsh et al 1993). Similar findings were obtained for the assessment of postoperative pain in dogs (Lascelles et al 1994). Comparisons of inter-observer variability using these scales has shown the agreement between observers using the SDS to be reasonable when assessing postoperative pain in dogs (Holton et al 1998), and the differences between two observers scoring lameness in sheep using the VAS or NRS were not significant (Welsh et al 1993). However, it has been suggested that the NRS may be the more suitable scale for assessing pain in a clinical setting, where a single knowledgeable person is responsible for pain management of the animal thoughout the perioperative period. It is possible that development of a multidimensional pain scoring system, which will be applicable to multicentre studies, may improve pain assessment techniques (Nolan & Reid, personal communication).

All of these pain scoring techniques rely primarily on behavioural signs, and interpretation of these is highly subjective. Detailed behavioural observations have been used to try to assess pain in both small laboratory mammals and farm

55

animals. Studies of the effects of tail docking and castration in lambs (Wood et al 1991, Mellor & Stafford 1999, Thornton & Waterman-Pearson 1999) and castration in piglets (McGlone & Hellman 1988) used a series of well-defined behavioural parameters to compare the effects of these husbandry procedures with and without the use of local anaesthetic. Control groups which underwent handling but no other procedure were also included. The behavioural analysis of lambs subjected to docking and castration showed a clear difference associated with the use of local anaesthetic, with animals behaving in a manner similar to those lambs which were only subjected to handling. The use of local anaesthetic to castrate piglets was also shown to have a significant effect.

Behavioural or action scoring is widely used in lameness assessment in horses. Diagnostic regional analgesia of the limbs is used throughout equine clinical practice to locate the site of pain causing the lameness; numerous means of quantifying the lamenesses are used, from a subjective score used for comparison by the same clinician after treatment to weight bearing as assessed by a force plate (Silver et al 1983, Schatzmann et al 1994). More sophisticated gait evaluation is also used through computer analysis of videotapes of horses moving on a treadmill (Clayton 1991). However, at present most biomechanical techniques are used for gait analysis and in experimental studies to assess potential forms of treatment (Keegan et al 1997) and as yet they are rarely used to assess the progress of clinical cases.

A few investigators have used scoring systems to assess the effects of a range of analgesics under clinical conditions in horses. Jochle et al (1989) used a range of behavioural and physiological signs to 'score' pain in horses with colic before and after administration of a number of analgesics. Most retrospective and some prospective studies of colic treatment and outcome use behavioural signs of pain as one of the criteria for classifying the severity of the disease (Ducharme et al 1989). There are very few studies investigating postoperative pain in horses. Johnson et al (1993) compared the effects of three NSAIDs after elective orthopaedic surgery using a score awarded by one of two assessors' subjective evaluation based on overall impression of behaviour. McCarthy et al (1993) attempted to use plasma β-endorphin measurement to assess pain and stress in horses but considered it too non-specific to be useful to aid clinical judgement. Raekallio et al (1997a, b) undertook two studies in an attempt to develop reliable methods of evaluating pain in horses in the way that has been achieved in dogs and laboratory mammals. Horses undergoing orthopaedic surgery were studied. A placebo controlled trial was conducted on horses undergoing arthroscopy (Raekallio et al 1997a) but horses undergoing more invasive surgery were all given analgesics (Raekallio et al 1997b). A number of behaviour patterns were assessed and endocrine and physiological changes were also recorded. Considerable difficulties were encountered in identifying useful objective measurements since few correlated with the predicted severity of pain. Hubbell (1999) has used a VAS in horses to assess the quality of recovery from anaesthesia and includes a VAS for pain. However, there are no published data validating the use of such a system in horses.

In laboratory animals, a number of different approaches have been used to assess pain or distress. The most extensive studies have been undertaken to investigate chronic pain, for example those by Colpaert et al (1980, 1982, 1987a), using an adjuvant arthritis model in the rat. Body weight, minute volume of respiration, mobility, vocalisations, specific behaviours and self-administration of analgesics were all considered as indices of pain. When discussing the results of all of these investigations, the authors concluded that all of the parameters responded to the same stimulus, and that the most reasonable explanation was that they were influenced by the presence of pain (Colpaert 1987). Motor behaviour changes have been suggested as indices of pain (Chudler & Dong 1983, Wright et al 1985) and loss of appetite and reduction in body weight have been noted in rodents postoperatively (Morton & Griffiths, 1985, Wright et al 1985, French et al 1986, 1988). These variables have been studied in rats as potential means of assessing the degree of postoperative pain, and of comparing the efficacy of different analgesic regimens (Flecknell & Liles 1991, 1992, Liles & Flecknell 1992a, 1993a, b, Liles et al 1997). Measures of food and water consumption and body weight are, of course, retrospective, and do not allow the analgesic regimen to be modified to meet the requirements of the individual animal. They do, however, enable broad assessments of analgesic efficacy to be made.

As with other pain assessment techniques in animals, most of the studies described above assume that if a change to a variable occurs after a procedure that would cause pain in man, then the change may be related to pain in the animal. If administration of an analgesic reverses these changes, this supports the hypothesis that the changes were, at least in part, pain related. This is a somewhat circular argument, since it is simply stating that indices of pain are those indices that are normalised by administration of analgesic drugs. Although efficacy of these analgesics in reducing peripheral nociceptive input in animals is well established (Crepax & Silvestrini 1963, Taber 1974, Albengres et al 1988, Kistler 1988), their effects on clinical pain are only validated in humans. Clearly, it is also important to establish that the analgesic does not have non-specific effects in normal animals that would influence the variable studied. Unfortunately, this has rarely been done in companion animals, so that many of the pain scoring systems could have been influenced by the side-effects of the analgesics used. Similarly, few studies in companion animals have compared scores in animals which have undergone surgery with those that have only been anaesthetised, although some studies have looked at indices such as plasma cortisol responses (Church et al 1994, Fox et al 1994). The importance of controlling for these effects has been demonstrated in rats, when the effects of buprenorphine on behaviour in normal animals prevented accurate assessment of its effects following surgery (Roughan & Flecknell 1997).

Critically, many investigators have felt it to be unethical to include a group of animals which undergo surgery without provision of an analgesic. The need for inclusion of a control group that undergoes surgery but receives no analgesic is clearly one that requires careful consideration. Many studies are undertaken in veterinary schools, where the standard practice for many years has been to assume that animals require pain relief following surgery, and therefore to administer analgesics. Nevertheless, if the pain scoring systems used are believed to be accurate and reliable, then it should be possible to devise a humane study which includes an untreated control group, but which incorporates intervention therapy if the pain score increases above a pre-defined threshold (Raekallio et al 1997a, b, Slingsby et al 1998, Firth & Haldane 1999, Lascelles et al 1998). It is also pertinent that routine clinical use of postoperative analgesia in animals is still far from widespread or uniform, and the information obtained from well-controlled clinical studies could be of considerable benefit to substantial numbers of animals. An alternative to use of a control group with intervention therapy would be to delay administration of the analgesic regimen until after full recovery from anaesthesia, as has been done in some studies of postoperative analgesia in children (McIlvaine et al 1988).

Manipulation pain

During clinical examination it is routine to use elicitation of pain as a marker of pathology, even if the animal has low grade chronic pain which is producing only subtle signs. This is done by palpation of the affected area or manipulation of the affected joint which exacerbates low grade pain to produce transient severe pain. While helpful in localising the problem, it is impossible to be sure that the intensity of the reaction to manipulation is truly representative of the severity of the pain felt by the animal in the absence of stimulation.

In summary, whether a scoring system is used or not, pain assessment will be facilitated by:

- A good knowledge of the species-specific behaviours of the animal being assessed
- A knowledge and comparison of the individual animal's behaviour before and after the onset of pain (e.g. pre- and postoperatively)
- The use of palpation or manipulation of the affected area and assessment of the responses obtained
- Examination of the level of function of the affected area, e.g. leg use following injury or limb surgery, together with a knowledge of any mechanical interference with function
- The use of analgesic regimens or dose rates that have been shown to be effective in controlled clinical studies, and evaluation of the change in behaviour this brings about
- A knowledge of the non-specific effects of any analgesic, anaesthetic or other drugs that have been administered.

Difficulties of assessing clinical pain

Most attempts to assess clinical pain employ behavioural observations, but many factors can influence behaviour, thus adding to our difficulties in interpreting how much pain an animal is experiencing.

Altered environment

Animals undergoing diagnosis and treatment of clinical disease are likely to be in a strange environment. Whatever the species, this may alter their normal behaviour and may mask signs of pain. The animals are likely to be apprehensive, nervous or excited. Animals that are adapted to disguise signs of ill health so they are not attacked by predators or herd members, e.g. some types of herbivore, may be especially difficult to assess, while dogs are often influenced by their desire to 'please' their human contact.

Animals that are normally herd animals, again particularly the herbivores, will be stressed by isolation from their peers and may not show overt signs of pain. Singleton neonates, especially, are less likely to show overt signs or vocalise as there are strong evolutionary disadvantages to this.

Pet animals are also affected by being in a strange environment; their normal territory is disrupted and strange smells and other animals may all be perceived as threatening. Dogs in particular may attempt to protect their owner – all leading to abnormal behaviour. The very presence or absence of the owner may also dramatically alter an animal's response to pain. The presence of other species may also alter the animal's responses. Cattle, sheep and rabbits will alter their behaviour in the presence of a predator (a dog, for example), minimising whatever subtle signs of pain they may be exhibiting. Cats may also change their behaviour dramatically in the presence of a dog.

Species differences

Interpretation of pain in a range of species depends on understanding the normal behaviour of each. For example, horses appear to experience greater pain than other species, if their dramatic responses to colic is contrasted with the behaviour of a cat that simply hides away after a road traffic accident. Presumably this is simply the individual's expression of pain, and does not accurately reflect the degree of pain it is experiencing. Behavioural effects can rarely be extrapolated from one species to another and attempts to anthropomorphise are fraught with problems. Individual species behaviour is described elsewhere in this chapter (see below).

Within-species variations

Even within a species, individual animals may respond to pain in very different ways. It is notable that different breeds of dogs may be stoical, such as the labrador, or 'wimpish,' such as the greyhound. Hence the former may run around and wag its tail even with a broken leg, while the greyhound will scream when given a subcutaneous vaccination. Which is experiencing the greater pain? Even within a breed, individual animals may react very differently. It is essential to get to know, as far as possible, the animal's normal behaviour before pain is assessed. In this respect, time spent with the animal is invaluable. It is also important to ask the owner and the nursing staff how the animal normally behaves.

The character and temperament of the animal will further influence its response. In any species, perhaps particularly in dogs, response to pain may be largely aggressive or defensive. Hence one dog may attempt to bite at a handler, another will try to escape or simply vocalise. A normally dominant dog is more likely to be aggressive when in pain while a quiet dog will often become more dull and anxious. The degree of pain experienced by the two animals may, however, be very similar.

Effect of other drugs

Many analgesics have sedative properties. Certainly, when they are used in association with anaesthesia for surgical treatment the effect may be to enhance sedation. However sedation does not necessarily indicate adequate analgesia and careful attempts to distinguish the two are necessary in ensuring that effective postoperative analgesia is provided. Opioids may also cause substantial changes in behaviour, e.g. increased or abnormal activity such as aimless walking, circling, head shaking, compulsive chewing and foot stamping. The particular responses seen vary considerably between species (see chapter 5).

Signs of pain in animals

All of the problems listed above need to be considered when trying to develop pain scoring systems. A final difficulty is that we are still unsure which types of behaviour best predict the severity of pain in different species. Nevertheless, we have attempted to describe the signs that we believe may be of value. These are quite detailed for the dog, cat and horse, but much less so for other species which have received less attention in relation to pain assessment and use of analgesics.

Signs of pain in dogs

Initial response to acute pain

Acute pain, such as that occurring during the actual process of tissue damage, will almost invariably produce an avoidance reaction in dogs. For minor injuries this may be minimal, e.g. the flinch down of the upper thoracic spine between the shoulder blades when a subcutaneous injection is made into the scruff is not usually considered to be a marker of great discomfort, but is nevertheless a sign that the dog has realised that an injury has occurred. Individuals vary in their reactions to minor injury, and some may vocalise. Facial expression may be unchanged, or there may be furrowing of the brows which appears to be a clear parallel to wincing, which is seen in humans. There may be minor attempts to distance themselves from the stimulus, e.g. by hiding behind their owner's legs, or there may be determined attempts to escape. In a small percentage of individuals what appears to be a trivial stimulus can provoke marked escape or aggressive behaviour.

The reaction to a simple injury can also be modified in many ways. Some dogs may show no reaction to a simple injection if distracted by a small morsel of food. Dogs which are well trained in obedience may sit immobile on command and this may override their natural avoidance reaction. Dogs which react with aggression may not be reacting to the pain *per se*, but rather to the perception that they are being attacked or threatened. The difference between the psychological insult and the physical injury is very obvious in dogs vaccinated by subcutaneous injection, which usually produces minor physical discomfort and minimal psychological disturbance, compared with those in which vaccine is administered intranasally. This latter route is almost certainly pain-free but frequently produces severe avoidance reactions, especially if the experience is repeated.

There are a number of procedures carried out on conscious dogs which appear to cause moderate pain. These include deep otoscopic examination of inflamed ear canals, emptying of inflamed anal sacs, nail paring which accidentally involves the sensitive vascular tissue, and removal of foreign bodies from infected sites such as interdigital abscesses. Although, as with responses to minor pain, there is marked individual variation, an individual is increasingly more likely to show an avoidance reaction as the severity of the pain increases. Very transient severe pain often elicits a vocalisation reaction, especially if the dog was not expecting the stimulus.

Severe pain is not normally deliberately inflicted on dogs, but in situations where this is unavoidable a spectrum of pain-related behaviours can be observed. For example, if a dog fractures a long bone, sustains a thermal injury, or is caught and dragged beneath a car, there is usually vocalisation, often at maximum volume, which persists for the duration of the trauma. This is accompanied by vigorous attempts to remove itself from the insult and from the location where it is occurring. Attempts to handle or restrain dogs in these situations will often be met with violent aggression. Even good-natured animals may behave completely out of character in such circumstances.

If the trauma is continuous, the initial increase in acute pain behaviours will be followed by an increased incidence of inactive behaviours and by apathy and depression, with recurrence of more active signs of pain if the dog is disturbed or tissue damage increases. Most animals undergoing surgery would experience this type of severe unremitting pain were they not rendered unconscious by anaesthesia. The other group of dogs which show signs of acute unremitting pain are those with neuropathic diseases, e.g. cervical spine disorders where there is repeated cord and nerve root compression and cervical muscle spasm.

Dogs with peripheral nerve injuries will frequently self-mutilate the affected limb. This can be seen occasionally following inadvertent sciatic nerve damage due to a migrating intramedullary pin and is probably analogous to autotomy in man (see chapter 7).

Additional responses to acute pain

Immediately following an injury there is a period of more or less severe pain for a variable period of time. Typically, the pain is most severe immediately following injury and subsides over several hours or days. A dog's reaction to this type of pain is also greatly influenced by temperament and the circumstances of the patient. Recovery from anaesthesia, when some degree of disorientation is present, is the time when marked vocalisation and attempts to escape are most likely to be seen. As recovery progresses and the animal recovers its coordination and awareness, whimpering is the more frequent type of vocalisation. Posture changes are used to minimise pressure on the affected area, and movement is often restricted. Recovery of consciousness is often faster in animals suffering from pain as the discomfort will mitigate against sleep. A patient which stands as soon as possible after laparotomy and subsequently refuses to sit or lie down is very likely to be in pain. In circumstances where the animal is able to reach the surgical site, such as after ear or eye surgery, pain will cause the patient to rub at the wound with its paws. Blepharospasm is a sign of ocular pain and head shaking is commonly indicative of ear pain. Rarely, mouth pain elicits a pawing reaction but most patients with pain after dental surgery do not paw at their mouths but will be depressed and dribble saliva. Body surface surgery which involves minimal deep tissue damage often causes little overt evidence of pain unless the wound is under tension. In these circumstances animals will often adopt a position which minimises skin tension once they are awake enough to behave in a coordinated manner.

Orthopaedic surgery will normally result in the affected limb being favoured, even though the mechanical problem with the limb has been corrected. Pain from orthopaedic surgery arises not only from the receptors in joints or periosteum but also from the soft tissue injury sustained during the surgery. In situations where pain is severe, such as may occur where a repair is unstable, where there has been peripheral nerve injury or where dressings are causing ischaemia, there will be persistent signs of severe pain with vocalisation, chewing at the dressings and marked restlessness. Limbs which are free to move may be held out sideways from the body, rigid and trembling, with the dog in lateral recumbency. Persistence of pain of this type will eventually lead to depression and lethargy, accompanied by withdrawal, aggression or comfort-seeking depending on the temperament of the dog.

Severe abdominal pain frequently results in depression, withdrawal and immobility. The muscles of the abdominal wall are tense and breathing is shallow to minimise diaphragmatic movement. Some dogs will persist in standing whereas others adopt a 'praying mantis' posture with elbows on the ground and hind limbs straight and weight bearing. Persistent abdominal pain in a sick animal that is sedated post-anaesthesia often results in the animal simply lying in sternal recumbency, moving as little as possible.

Injury to the sacrococcygeal junction is quite common in dogs and typically results in a hanging tail which the dog wags as little as possible. Lively dogs are frequently reported as being very subdued with this type of injury. Surgery to the distal tail, especially amputation, appears to produce repeated bouts of pain when the dog will suddenly jump and chew at the surgical site.

Post-injury pain

As time passes after acute injury and as dogs recover from the behavioural effects of general anaesthesia they show fewer overt signs of pain. When the animal is returned to their owner, it may well be distracted and this will mask the more subtle signs of pain. Once settled again, however, whimpering will indicate pain and direct trauma to the surgical site will often elicit vocalisation and avoidance behaviour. Low grade pain is most clearly demonstrated by a reluct-ance to move. If a dog perceives that movement increases its pain it is well able to restrict its own activity. Loss of appetite, especially in a dog which normally eats well, can be a marker of ongoing pain, especially if any anaesthetic which has been given is one which usually results in rapid recovery. Moderate pain will not usually stop the essential survival behaviour of eating, but food intake may be reduced. Although some dogs will chew at comfortable wound dressings, those which persistently attempt to remove their dressings may well have localised pain.

Chronic pain

Acute pain is generally related to specific tissue damage and resolves as the dam-age resolves. Chronic pain is a distinct entity and may be present in the absence of obvious tissue pathology. In addition, the severity of the pain may not correl-ate with the severity of any pathology which is present. For example, dogs with chronic osteoarthritis may have differing degrees of pain (lameness) with similar degrees of pathology. Chronic pain, especially if insidious in onset, may well go unnoticed in dogs, even by their owners. Dogs with severe osteoarthritic pain may be described as having stiffness, or problems with getting up, especially after periods of recumbency. If their problems are symmetrical they may have a short-stepping or 'doddery' gait. Bilateral hind limb pain will cause the dog to arch its spine and transfer as much weight as possible onto its front legs. Similar gait changes are also seen with thoracolumbar or lumbar spinal pain. Also associated with chronic lack of function, but not indicating pain *per se*, is muscle atrophy on the affected leg. If there is no neurological explanation the assumption must be that the disuse which leads to atrophy is caused by pain. Subtle changes such as decreased toe-nail wear may also indicate chronic pain in a given limb.

Pain caused by dental disease may also result in relatively subtle signs, such as the uneven development of plaque and tartar where the condition is unilateral, with most plaque forming on the side which causes discomfort when the dog chews.

A number of dogs with severe persistent pain such as is associated with moderate spinal cord compression will show a marked decrease in their interest in life, and decreased appetite. Dogs with low grade osteoarthritis may be reluctant to climb stairs, jump into cars and may show reduced levels of activity. All are indicators of chronic pain. A retrospective assessment of the degree of pain experienced in all of these circumstances is to observe the change in demeanour after administration of an analgesic agent, which will often dramatically improve activity levels back towards normal.

Signs of pain in cats

Initial response to acute pain

The reflex response to minor trauma while it is occurring includes flinching, a short cry or growl, cowering and occasional aggression with variable attempts to escape. The response to ongoing severe injury in cats is hissing and spitting, vigorous attempts to escape and marked aggression. As in other species, if the trauma is continuous the overt typical response may eventually be replaced by depression and apathy unless a change in the intensity or nature of the trauma occurs.

Additional responses to acute pain

Immediately after minor trauma a cat's behaviour may not alter in any obvious way, or it may become aggressive, or attempt to find a safe hiding place. These responses are subject to marked individual variation. A number of cats will adopt a hunched position with head down, shoulders lowered and elbows out following the injection of irritant drugs into their scruff. Intramuscular injections, particularly of irritant drugs into limb muscles, will often produce a reduction in weight bearing on the damaged leg for a variable period of time depending upon the site used, the irritancy of the drug and its proximity to major nerve trunks.

In the aftermath of major trauma cats are usually depressed, immobile, silent, and will appear tense and distanced from their environment. Vocalisation is rare except for the occasional low growl. After major trauma cats will also hyperventilate. This frequently responds to analgesic therapy, suggesting it is a pain-related behaviour.

Very occasionally after major surgery cats will recover from anaesthesia and demonstrate a manic reaction of aggression and rolling around their cage. If pain from limb surgery is severe it can result in cats attacking their dressings or attempting to 'throw' the operated limb/dressing away. This can be accompanied by marked vocalisation. After abdominal surgery cats in pain adopt sternal recumbency, keep their elbows well back, stifles well forward and tense their abdominal muscles. Their facial expression is anxious. Pain after facial trauma often results in the cat appearing depressed and adopting a head down, face down position. Nasal, ocular and anal pain often results in attempts to rub or scratch the affected area. If pain is severe, self-mutilation can result.

Later in the time course following major injury, cats exhibit marked withdrawal. For example, after a road traffic accident a cat may fail to return home, and instead find a secluded location where it may stay for several days. In cats which are confined in a kennel or at home a withdrawal reaction still frequently occurs, with some individuals seeking hiding places under furniture or in cupboards. Vocalisation at this stage is very rare, but depression and anorexia or decreased appetite are common.

Chronic pain

There are few specific signs of persistent low grade pain in cats. Lack of activity, decreased interest in their surroundings and weight loss due to inappetence or reduced food and water consumption may all be noted. Localised pain can produce more specific signs such as slow or one-sided eating with dental pain. This is often not recognised as pain until the dental problem is corrected, when the cat's owner will frequently report improved well-being in addition to improved appetite. Single joint orthopaedic pain will be exhibited as lameness, stiffness after rest and muscle wastage on the affected leg. Multiple joint pain often causes a decrease in activity, increased stiffness and a short stepping or crouching gait.

Signs of pain in horses

There are remarkably few reports describing methods of 'objective' assessment of pain in horses (Raekallio 1997a, b, Hubbell 1999). However, this species exhibits a number of behavioural characteristics that are widely accepted as evidence that the horse is experiencing pain.

The horse is essentially a 'flight' animal and commonly its reaction to any stimulus that frightens or hurts it is to attempt to escape from the source. It may then be difficult to distinguish whether it is experiencing pain or another unpleasant sensation. A horse may respond violently to a relatively innocuous touch, sometimes making it difficult to distinguish pain from other behavioural problems.

Acute pain

Sharp, sudden onset pain usually induces a reflex escape or attack reaction. Hence a horse may gallop off or move away or alternatively may kick or bite at the source of the stimulus. For instance, an insect bite usually elicits a kick or bite at the affected area; if this does not dislodge the offending arthropod a horse may gallop off, or if in a restricted area become restless and excited.

Head pain elicits head shaking, snorting and restlessness. If associated with mouth or jaw pain, difficulty in eating may be noted, with drooling of saliva and chewing confined to one side of the jaw. Limb pain leads to stamping and constant picking up and replacement of the limb. Alternatively the limb may be held on the ground but the weight taken off the heel or occasionally the toe. Abdominal pain causes general restlessness, kicking at the belly, glancing at the flanks and rolling. Tail swishing in the absence of any other cause, such as flies, is often a sign of pain and is often seen when pain is severe enough to make the horse restless and distressed. Behaviour in response to pain may become extremely abnormal: a general restlessness and jerky movement, where the horse moves forwards a few strides, stops, swishes its tail and lowers and possibly shakes its head, followed by a further few strides forwards is often seen in response to sudden onset, intermittent pain. This is particularly associated with relatively mild pain, e.g. after nettle sting.

Unrelenting/severe pain

More severe and unrelenting pain leads to some of the behaviour described above but it is persistent, distinctly giving the impression that although the pain may vary in severity, it is continuous. Horses with severe pain, whatever the source, are restless, tachypnoeic, tachycardiac, agitated and sweat copiously. Since equine sweat has a high protein content it may appear as foam on the neck and flanks. The horse's attitude changes and it may become difficult to communicate with, adopts a wild and distracted appearance to the eye and takes little care to avoid knocking into a person or other animal. Some horses may snatch at food, take a mouthful, fail to chew on it but return for another snatched mouthful. Some will play with drinking water but do not swallow any.

In addition to the general signs of severe pain, colic causes distracted kicking at the belly, glancing at the flank and repeatedly lying down, rolling and getting up again. Sometimes the horse may stay in lateral or partial dorsal recumbency for a few minutes, in an abnormal, hunched or stretched posture before getting up again. The horse may stretch out as though to urinate but produce little or no urine. Throughout this restlessness, the horse sweats, sometimes copiously until it becomes dehydrated. Horses with colic may repeatedly go to the drinking water, sometimes taking a few mouthfuls or standing over the bucket and splashing water around as described above. Some horses with abdominal pain will even snatch at food. Lip curling is also seen.

Severe limb pain causes marked lameness and constant lifting of the leg, touching it down and lifting it again. Restlessness, agitation and sweating are marked. Occasionally, immediately after an injury such as a fracture, the horse may continue to gallop, even jump or graze for some time. This appears similar to the well-known effect sometimes seen in man after traumatic injury during physical combat (so called 'battlefield analgesia') in that no pain is experienced at the time of injury and may not develop until some hours later.

Severe pain affecting more than one limb, e.g. laminitis, leads to a very different picture. Sweating, tachypnoea and dyspnoea are present but the animal develops a fixed, board-like posture and is reluctant to move. It may be difficult to distinguish from colic in some instances.

Severe head pain may progress from head shaking to a lowered head and head pressing, and eventually to extreme depression.

Chronic pain

Persistent pain eventually leads to the horse appearing depressed, standing with its head down, avoiding other horses or standing in the corner of the stable. Tension in abdominal muscles may give a tucked up appearance. Back and neck pain may lead to abnormal head and neck posture, sometimes with the head held to one side, or tilted. Mental alertness is decreased and the eye appears dull, listless and distant. There is no interest in food or water and the horse may spend long periods lying down. Severe colic is unlikely to progress in this way as the condition eliciting the pain is likely to be fatal before this stage is reached. However, laminitis, peritonitis and rhabdomyolysis may all cause such depression.

Other species

Less information is available concerning pain behaviour in other species, although pain behaviour in certain specific situations in cattle, sheep and rats has been studied (see below). Most of the mammalian species show similar immediate responses to an acute painful stimulus. This is usually escape behaviour, sometimes coupled with aggression, and vocalisation. Pain in localised areas, e.g. the limbs, results in lameness. Ocular pain usually causes blepharospasm and guarding behaviour, although this is not always seen in small mammals. Further information for each species is given below.

Pain in cattle, sheep and goats

Ruminant species are prey species and so there are good evolutionary reasons why they tend not to exhibit overt behavioural signs of pain. Obvious behavioural cues would mark an individual out and make it more likely to be the target of a predator in the wild. The signs of pain in these species are therefore subtle, but just because they do not show marked active behavioural signs does not mean that they do not suffer pain just as intensely as other species.

The behavioural cues shown by these animals vary with the type and severity of the pain which is present. Overt behavioural changes in cattle, e.g. aggression to conspecifics or even to man, should alert one to the possibility that the animal is suffering from a neurological disorder such as BSE or listeria. Neurological disorders will give rise to a variety of signs such as aggression, head pressing and teeth grinding in all three of the species.

Cattle

Pain of visceral origin (abdominal or thoracic) is characterised by total or partial inappetence, dullness, depression and increased respiratory rate, with abdominal splinting and grunting being especially evident. Severe pain may actually lead to bellowing, teeth grinding, and cessation of rumination and cudding. Visceral pain is accompanied by tachycardia and other sympathetic mediated changes. As the severity of the pain increases cattle are more and more reluctant to move and will also resort to flank kicking, but this behaviour does not develop into the uncontrolled behaviour seen in horses. Cattle with abdominal pain may also repeatedly lie down and then stand again, or may remain recumbent. More prolonged pain can result in the animal becoming separated from the rest of the herd, if group housed.

Upper abdominal pain is a cardinal sign of traumatic reticuloperitonitis and may be elicited by positioning a pole under the anterior abdomen. A brisk upwards press elicits a marked grunt response indicative of reticulitis and post-thoracic abscessation.

Lameness is a major welfare problem in cattle and sheep and pain associated with localised orthopaedic conditions is most commonly manifest as lameness. However, it should be emphasised that if the animal has lesions in more than one hind limb then the lameness may not be very obvious at first glance, although careful examination will reveal a stilted gait and arching of the back as the cow attempts to throw her weight forward on to her forelimbs. Reluctance to move will predispose to reduced body condition as the animal will be less able to compete for food at feeding.

Chronic pain leads to reduced grooming behaviour in cattle; this is apparent with both low grade visceral and somatic pain. Localised sites of pain will give rise to specific pain behaviours, e.g. lacrimation and blepharospasm are obviously cues that the animal is suffering ocular discomfort. Mastitis will cause pain such that the cow may show allodynia, resenting handling of the inflamed mammary gland as merely touching becomes painful. Straining is an obvious indicator of pain that may be associated with either the urinary tract (obstruction or inflammation) or the genital tract.

Sheep

Sheep are similar to cattle in some respects; they are very prone to foot-rot and the pain associated with this disease gives rise to progressive lameness. Sheep with severe foot-rot will tend to graze on their knees in order to reduce the pain associated with weight bearing. They will also tend to lose body condition. Visceral pain tends to be more difficult to detect than in cattle. Sheep will grind their teeth and curl their lips and will stop cudding, but they do not tend to grunt or vocalise.

Sheep will exhibit both teeth grinding and head pressing when in severe pain. After traumatic injury, sheep may show few overt signs of pain, but careful observation by an experienced clinician or animal handler can often detect subtle changes in demeanour that are associated with the presence of pain. Chronic pain leads to loss of condition and general dullness.

Goats

Goats are much more demonstrative than sheep. If they are in pain they will stop grooming and resent handling. They are very vocal animals and acute pain will evoke a marked increase in bleating and crying. Visceral pain will give rise to the same signs as seen in cattle (cessation of cudding, inappetence, flank watching and kicking, tachycardia, increased respiratory rate with splinting).

Pain behaviours elicited by castration/tail docking

Lambs and probably calves and goat kids have a limited repertoire of behaviours that they can employ to indicate their needs. Thus these young animals are more vocal than adults. Pain associated with husbandry procedures such as castration will cause marked changes in behaviour patterns.

Depending on the method of castration employed, lambs show a range of behavioural changes. Following application of rubber rings, when there is longer term but slightly less acute pain, lambs show an increase in active behaviours, with general restlessness and adoption of abnormal postures such as statue standing, dog sitting and tail wagging; foot stamping and rolling, flank kicking and lying laterally with hind legs extended backwards may occur. In contrast, following surgical castration, when there is much more severe acute pain, there is an increase in passive behaviours, with lambs moving less and more likely to be recumbent. Older lambs show less active pain behaviours following castration, indicating that the overt signs of pain will change as animals develop and mature. Lambs show reduced feeding activity for some 24 hours post-castration. Although these acute signs of pain abate within eight hours or so, lambs will show marked reduced playing behaviour for some three days post-castration, suggesting that they continue to suffer pain for at least this period. Calves and lambs spend more time lying laterally following castration and both lambs and piglets exhibit tail wagging following docking.

Pain in pigs

Pigs tend normally to resent handling but paradoxically when they are in pain they will often tolerate handling more readily. When experiencing prolonged acute pain, e.g. following surgery, pigs may be reluctant to stand, and move slowly, if at all. Pigs will often become completely inappetent when in pain, although some animals will continue to eat. Animals may play with their water bowls or drinker spouts, but not actually swallow any water. Although pigs have few muscles of facial expression, there are subtle changes in appearance, particularly in relation to the position of the eye with increased tension in the periocular area. Acute pain tends to provoke shivering and piloerection and pigs subjected to the stress of transport may often suffer from travel sickness.

When suffering from abdominal pain, e.g. after abdominal surgery, they may lie with their hind limbs extended, with tensed abdominal muscles. Palpation of the abdomen can cause the pig to vocalise. In adults this is usually grunting, but short higher pitched sounds may be made. When being encouraged to move, the animal may vocalise repeatedly, either aggressively with repeated short grunts or at a higher pitch. This latter sound is usually very different from the loud squealing that occurs when pigs are being handled or fed. When encouraged to walk, the animal may have an abnormal gait, often with a 'tucked up' appearance to the abdomen. When experiencing pain they may become passive and apathetic, and be almost completely unresponsive to stimuli, which is unusual as pigs normally resent handling and avoid it. Limb pain is usually associated with lameness, and is relatively easy to detect, although it is not always easy to elicit a response when palpating the limb.

Any unexplained changes in behaviour should alert the stockman to the possibility that the animal is in pain. As with most farm species, chronic pain associated with lameness will lead to weight loss as the animal is less able to compete for food.

Pain in small rodents and rabbits

Pain is more difficult to assess in these small mammals than in cats and dogs. This is primarily because the behaviours associated with pain are more subtle, and also because as clinicians we are less familiar with the normal appearance and behaviour of these species. The immediate response to acute pain is similar to other species. The animal attempts to remove itself from the source of the painful stimulus, it may vocalise, and it may show aggressive behaviour, especially if it is unable to escape from the stimulus (e.g. when being restrained for an injection). When experiencing severe pain, rabbits may squeal, but this seems more often to be in response to fear. Following accidental injury or surgical trauma, most small mammals reduce their overall level of spontaneous activity. Both rabbits and small rodents may become completely immobile when experiencing moderate to severe postoperative pain, and will usually position themselves in the furthest corner of a recovery box, or may try to hide under bedding or under a food hopper. The animal usually remains immobile even when approached, but may attempt to escape when handled. When moving, the animal's gait may be altered, and it may show a reduced frequency of behaviours such as grooming or rearing, but detecting this requires careful observation by a trained observer. Rats show a characteristic stretching and back-arching behaviour following abdominal surgery, and may press their abdomens onto the ground. They also show frequent sudden short movements while resting.

Rodents may become unusually aggressive when handled, and may vocalise, sometimes at an abnormal pitch. It is important to remember that these species may vocalise at a frequency which is outside the range of human hearing. Observing the behaviour of small mammals can be difficult as some species are nocturnal (e.g. rat, hamster, gerbil) and so will be relatively inactive during the day. In addition, they often change their behaviour in the presence of an observer. This is particularly noticeable with rabbits and guinea pigs, who may become completely immobile.

In addition to changes in behaviour, the animal's external appearance may be altered, e.g. small rodents may show a hunched up posture. In addition, they may show piloerection, and soiling of the coat indicating lack of grooming. Grooming can be reduced in all species, and in rats this can lead to build up of reddish brown secretions around the eyes and nose. This material is porphyrin, excreted from the harderian glands. This appearance is a non-specific stress response, but should alert the clinician to the possibility that the stress involved may be pain. When housed in small groups, rats, mice, guinea pigs and rabbits may separate themselves from their cage or pen mates when they are in pain. As with other species, abdominal pain can cause tensing of the abdomen in rabbits, with a 'tucked up' appearance to the abdomen. Rabbits with abdominal pain may also grind their teeth.

Small rodents and rabbits often show reduced appetite if pain is not alleviated effectively. This reduction may go unnoticed if the animal is fed *ad lib* and has a large water bowl or bottle, but can often be detected as a fall in body weight. The quantity of faeces and urine produced will also be reduced, but this can be difficult to detect in small rodents. These reductions in food intake are particularly important in rabbits and guinea pigs, as they can trigger gastrointestinal disturbances that can prove fatal. Although rodents and rabbits may show changes in the pattern and depth of respiration and in heart rate, the normal responses to handling may mask these alterations.

As with other species, many of the changes described above are not associated only with the presence of pain, and must be interpreted together with the clinical history of the animal. Administering an analgesic may be of help in confirming that pain is the cause of the changes.

Pain in non-mammalian species

There is a significant increase in the number of non-mammalian animals being presented to veterinary surgeons. Certain avian species such as poultry, parrots, small cage birds and pigeons have been veterinary patients for some time. However the majority of pharmacological interventions have focussed on treatment of infection and infestations and the provision of anaesthesia. It is only in recent years that control of pain has been addressed.

Pain in birds

Responses to acute pain are often even more subtle in birds than in mammals. This can lead to an assumption that they experience less pain. However, the neuroanatomical mechanisms for nociception are present in birds. They possess μ, κ and δ opioid receptors and α-2 binding sites in their brains (Danbury et al 1998a) and also possess ORL1 receptors and I2 binding sites. Nociceptin (orphanin FQ) has been proposed as the endogenous opioid for the novel orphan receptor ORL1. This receptor and its ligand seem to play a role in nociption although its exact role is as yet unclear. The receptor has previously been shown to exist in rats, rabbits and guinea pigs, but had not been investigated in chickens. Its finding in addition to μ, δ and κ binding sites in chickens lends further support to the contention that chickens have the same capacity to perceive pain as mammals – and also that opioids are likely to be good analgesics. The proportion of receptor subtypes is remarkably close to those in man (23% μ, 30% δ, 26% κ, 20% ORL1). Chickens have also been shown to have α-2 receptors mapped closely to the distribution in mammals – and there was upregulation in lame birds in the locus coerulus and raphe nucleus (Danbury et al 1998a and b, Danbury et al 1999, Danbury 1999). Studies in poultry (McGeown et al 1999) and parrots (Paul-Murphy 1998) have been published recently, indicating that pain assessment and assessment of analgesic efficacy can be undertaken in these species. The presence of nociceptors in chickens has been demonstrated, but the clinical responses of birds to noxious stimuli vary considerably (Gentle 1992).

Acute pain in birds

Mild pain may elicit vocalisation (in some species of birds) and wing flapping which can progress to droop. Birds will also tend to show increased respiratory rate and often will 'mouth breathe' when distressed, and their feathers become ruffled. This ruffled appearance may be exacerbated by lack of preening, although a localised painful area may be preened excessively, resulting in localised feather loss. If the source of pain is localised, birds may show guarding behaviour and may not use the affected body part. Severe distress triggers a catatonic reaction in birds, presumably a survival mechanism, when they become immobile and totally unresponsive. More prolonged or less severe pain can produce behavioural changes such as decreased activity, lack of social interactions with other birds or the owner, and decreased appetite and consequent weight loss.

Chronic pain in birds

Pain in birds has been studied most comprehensively in broiler chickens. Broilers are the most numerous farmed species, with some 40 billion produced per annum worldwide. Genetic selection has led to greatly increased growth rates with slaughter weight being reached when the skeleton is still very immature. This has led to an increase in lameness as a host of pathologies cause a progressive degree of pain and impaired walking ability. The severity of lameness ranges from slight lameness to inability to walk without using their wings to balance. Lame birds spend a large proportion of their time lying down, often with one leg held extended. They eat less often and may choose to eat lying down. Evidence that they are in pain is reinforced by a reduction in the time they spend preening and dust bathing compared to sound birds. Birds with long term pain also exhibit wing droop.

Recent studies using analgesics as an experimental tool have confirmed that lame birds are in pain, since analgesics significantly improve their walking ability in an obstacle test, and lame birds will choose to eat food containing analgesics, while sound birds do not, suggesting that the drugs alleviate an unpleasant sensation (Danbury et al 2000).

Mutilations such as debeaking also offer insights into the pain suffered by birds. Normally, birds use their beaks not just for eating but also for investigating their environment. When debeaked, this latter use ceases suggesting that the tip of the amputated beak develops allodynia or even neuropathic pain sensations.

Pain in fish, amphibia and reptiles

As discussed above, little is known concerning pain behaviour in non-mammalian species. It is clear that fish, reptiles and amphibia all show avoidance reactions to acute noxious stimuli, and this has been well documented in some amphibia (Stevens 1992, Stevens & Kirkendall 1992, Stevens et al 1994, Stevens & Roth 1997) and there is some information in reptiles (crocodiles: Kanui & Hole 1992). Noxious stimuli such as electric shock have been used in laboratory studies to modify behaviour in fish. Some of the more primitive fish, such as holosteans, have been used as electrophysiological models and nociceptive reflexes have been recorded (Martin & Wickelgren 1971). Teleosts are relatively neglected. Analgesia testing in fish has been restricted to assessing the effects of morphine in goldfish (Jansen & Greene 1970) and the effects of morphine antagonists (Ehrensing et al 1982) using an electrical stimulus. Other methods using thermal or mechanical stimuli appear not to have been used in fish.

Teleosts, in particular trout and salmon, are being farmed in ever greater numbers and are being subjected to greater contact with man than before. Intensive farming often results in disease or injury which in mammals would be assumed to be painful. In mammals, slaughter techniques are designed to avoid pain and suffering but it is not known if fish feel pain or even if they have the necessary neural structures.

The Institute of Medical Ethics has attempted to define a number of criteria to assess if an animal is capable of feeling pain (Smith & Boyd 1991). These fall into two categories:

- The animal must have similar anatomical and physiological mechanisms to those involved in pain perception in man (nociceptors, transmission neurones, thalamus and cortex, or their homologues)
- The animal must display analogous behaviour in response to pain and analgesic drugs which are effective in humans.

One of the criteria is the presence of opioid receptors. Although the major function of these in mammals is the modulation of pain, this may be an evolutionary adaptation, as they are also involved in a number of other roles such as reproduction (Rosenblum & Peter 1989) and are phylogenetically well conserved (Pert et al 1974). In recent years the number of neurotransmitters known to be involved with pain processing in mammals has increased enormously, but nothing is known of their role in fish.

Studies of clinical pain are completely lacking in fish, amphibia and reptiles, so virtually no information is available concerning appropriate dose rates of analgesic drugs, although some suggestions have been made based on clinical experience, and these are included in Tables 5.5 and 5.9 (chapter 5). At present, all that can be suggested for clinicians is that they should consider the possibility that pain could be present when dealing with these species, and that animals are observed carefully for any behavioural signs that could indicate pain.

Non-mammalian analgesia

One point which does seem to come up in the studies of non-mammalian vertebrates is the nature of the behavioural response to pain. While this will obviously take different forms in different species, as it does in mammals, there does seem to be less of a gradation in response. While this may only reflect the inadequacy of the testing methods, it may reflect a difference in the level of neuronal integration. Basically, the responses to painful stimuli seem to be more of an 'on–off' nature. What is also interesting, is that this can also be seen in the efficacy of the analgesic response, where there seems to be a steep dose–response curve, indicating that at a particular dose there will be either a good analgesic effect or none. Perhaps these observations reflect only the lack of sensitivity of the test system, possibly from attempting to transfer 'mammalian derived' tests to non-mammalian species, or perhaps this is a genuine difference from mammals. There are some reviews available; however, they are often found in unusual journals or some specific texts (Stoskopf 1994, Bennet 1998, Clyde & Paul-Murphy 1998, Machin 1999).

There is also considerable interest in invertebrate species and their perception of pain. While they all show varying degrees of avoidance behaviour to noxious stimuli and may well show learning abilities associated with this, there are very few data available to allow us to debate the concept of pain as we understand it in vertebrates. Opioid receptors have been demonstrated in non-vertebrates, but their function has not been accurately defined. So, as yet, the jury is out, but we must remember that some species can show sophisticated and integrative behaviour, e.g. the octopi and other higher molluscs, and also some of the more active crustacea and insects. The other important thing to remember is that a single order of the invertebrates may show more diversity than *all* of the vertebrates, and so there is unlikely to be a simple single answer to the question, 'Do invertebrates feel pain?'.

References

Albengres, E., Pinquier, J.L., Riant, P., et al (1988) Pharmacological criteria for risk-benefit evaluation of NSAIDs. *Scandinavian Journal of Rheumatology* **73** (Suppl): 3–15.

Anand, K. (1990) The biology of pain perception in newborn infants. *Advances in Pain Research and Therapy* **15**: 113–122.

Anand, K., Sippell, W.G., Aynsley-Green, A. (1987) Randomised trial of fentanyl anaesthesia in preterm babies undergoing surgery: effects on the stress response. *Lancet* (January): 243–249.

Bennett, R.A. (1998) Pain and analgesia in reptiles and amphibians. *Proceedings of the American Association of Zoological Veterinarians and American Association of Wildlife Veterinarians Joint Conference* pp. 461–465.

Chudler, E.H. and Dong, W.K. (1983) Neuroma pain model: correlation of motor behavior and body weight with autotomy in rats. *Pain* **17**: 341–351.

Church, D.B., Nicholson, A.I., Ilkiw, J.E., Emslie, D.R. (1994) Effect of non-adrenal illness, anaesthesia and surgery on plasma cortisol concentrations in dogs. *Research in Veterinary Science* **56**: 129–131.

Clayton, H.M. (1991) Advances in motion analysis. *Veterinary Clinics of North America Equine Practice* 7(**2**): 365–382.

Clyde, V.L. and Paul-Murphy, J. (1998) Avian analgesia. In: Fowler, M.E. and Miller, R.E. (eds) *Zoo and Wild Animal Medicine – Current Therapy*. W.B. Saunders Co., Philadelphia, ch. 39, pp. 309–314.

Colpaert, F.C. (1987) Evidence that adjuvant arthritis in the rat is associated with chronic pain. *Pain* **28**: 201–222.

Colpaert, F.C., DeWitte, P., Maroli, A.N., Awouters, F., Niemegeers, C.J.E. and Janssen, P.A.J. (1980) Self-administration of the analgesic suprofen in arthritic rats: evidence of *Mycobacterium butyricum* induced arthritis as an experimental model of chronic pain. *Life Sciences* **27**: 921–928.

Colpaert, F.C., Meert, T., DeWitte, P. and Schmitt, P. (1982) Further evidence validating adjuvant arthritis as an experimental model of chronic pain in the rat. *Life Sciences* **31**: 67–75.

Colpaert, F., Bervoets, K.J.W. and VandenHoogen, R.H.W.M. (1987a) Pharmacological analysis of hyperventilation in arthritic rats. *Pain* **30**: 243–258.

Conzemius, M.G., Hill, C.M., Sammarco, J.L. and Perkowski, S.Z. (1997) Correlation between subjective and objective measures used to determine severity of post-operative pain in dogs. *Journal of the American Veterinary Medical Association* **210**: 1619–1622.

Crepax, P. and Silvestrini, B. (1963) Experimental evaluation in laboratory animals of anti-inflammatory analgesic drugs. *Archives of Italian Biology* **101**: 444–457.

Danbury, T.C., Huson, A.L., Waterman-Pearson, A.E., Henderson, G. and Kestin, S.C. (1998a) Saturation binding of μ, δ and κ opioid ligands in chicken brains. *Archives of Pharmacology* **358**, **1** (suppl): 35. 105.

Danbury, T.C., Ruban, B., Hudson, A.L., Waterman-Pearson, A.E. and Kestin, S.C. (1998b) Imadzoline 2 binding sites in chicken brain. *Annals of New York Academy of Science* **881**: 189–192.

Danbury, T.C. (1999) Pain associated with lameness in broiler chickens: a behavioural and pharmacological study. PhD thesis. University of Bristol, Bristol, pp 165–210.

Danbury, T.C., Weeks, C., Kestin, S.C. and Waterman-Pearson, A.E. (2000) Self-selection of the analgesic drug carprofen by lame broiler chickens. *Veterinary Record* **146**: 307–311.

Ducharme, N.G., Pascoe, P.J., Lumsden, J.H. and Ducharme, G.R. (1989) A computer derived model to aid in selecting medical versus surgical treatment of horses with abdominal pain. *Equine Veterinary Journal* **21**: 447–450.

Ehrensing, R.H., Michell, G.F. and Kastin, A.J. (1982) Similar antagonism of morphine analgesia by MIF-1 and naloxone in *Carassius auratus*. *Pharmacology, Biochemistry and Behaviour* **17**: 757–761.

Firth, A.M. and Haldane, S.L. (1999) Development of a scale to evaluate postoperative pain in dogs. *Journal of the American Veterinary Medical Association* 214(**5**): 651–659.

Flecknell, P.A. (1984) The relief of pain in laboratory animals. *Laboratory Animals* **18**: 147–160.

Flecknell, P.A. (1994) Advances in the assessment and alleviation of pain in laboratory and domestic animals. *Journal of Veterinary Anaesthesia* **21**: 98–105.

Flecknell, P.A. and Liles, J.H. (1991) The effects of surgical procedures, halothane anaesthesia and nalbuphine on the locomotor activity and food and water consumption in rats. *Laboratory Animals* **25**: 50–60.

Flecknell, P.A. and Liles, J.H. (1992) Evaluation of locomotor activity and food and water consumption as a method of assessing postoperative pain in rodents. In: Short, C.E. and VanPoznak, A. (eds) *Animal Pain*. Churchill Livingstone, New York, pp 482–488.

Fox, S.M., Mellor, D.J., Firth, E.C., Hodge, H. and Lawoko, C.R.O. (1994) Changes in plasma cortisol concentrations before, during and after analgesia, anaesthesia and anaethesia plus ovario-hysterectomy in bitches. *Research in Veterinary Science* **57**: 110–118.

French, T.J., Goode, A.W., Schofield, P.S. and Sugden, M.C. (1986) Effects of surgical stress on the response of hepatic carnitine metabolism to 48 h starvation in the rat. *Biochimica et Biophysica Acta* **883**: 396–399.

French, T.J., Holness, M.J., Goode, A.W. and Sugden, M.C. (1988) Acute effects of surgery on carbohydrate production and utilization in the fed rat. *Clinical Science* **74**: 107–112.

Gentle, M.J. (1992) Pain in birds. *Animal Welfare* **1**: 235–247.

Holton, L.L., Scott, E.M., Nolan, A.M., Reid, J., Welsh, E. and Flaherty, D. (1998) Comparison of three methods used for assessment of pain in dogs. *Journal of the American Veterinary Medical Association* 212(**1**): 61–66.

Hubbell, J.A.E. (1999) Recovery from anaesthesia in horses. *Equine Veterinary Education* **11**: 160–167.

Jansen, G.A. and Greene, N.M. (1970) Morphine metabolism and morphine tolerance in goldfish. *Anesthesiology* **32**: 231–235.

Jochle, W., Moore, J.N., Brown, J., et al (1989) Comparison of detomidine, butorphanol, flunixine meglamine and xylazine in clinical cases of equine colic. *Equine Veterinary Journal* **7** (Suppl): 111–116.

Johnson, C.B., Taylor, P.M., Young, S.S. and Brearley, J.C. (1993) Postoperative analgesia using phenylbutazone, flunixin or carprofen in horses. *Veterinary Record* **133**: 336–338.

Kamerling, S., Wood, T., DeQuick, D., et al (1989) Narcotic analgesics, their detection and pain measurement in the horse: a review. *Equine Veterinary Journal* 21(**1**): 4–12.

Kanui, T.I. and Hole, K. (1992) Morphine and pethidine antinociception in the crocodile. *Journal of Veterinary Pharmacology and Therapeutics* **15**: 101–103.

Keegan, K.G., Wilson, D.J., Wilson, D.A., Frankeny, R.L., Loch, W.E. and Smith, B. (1997) Effects of anesthesia of the palmar digital nerves on kinematic gait analysis in horses with and without navicular disease. *American Journal of Veterinary Research* March, 58(**3**): 218–223.

Kistler, P. (1988) Zur Schmerzbekampfung im Tierversuch (Attenuation of pain in animal experimentation). PhD thesis, Bern.

Lascelles, B.D.X. (1996) Recent advances in the control of pain in animals. In: Raw, M.E. and Parkinson, T. (eds) *The Veterinary Annual*. Blackwell Science, Oxford, pp 1–16.

Lascelles, B.D.X., Butterworth, S.J. and Waterman, A.E. (1994) Post-operative analgesic and sedative effects of carprofen and pethidine in dogs. *Veterinary Record* **134**: 187–191.

Lascelles, B.D.X., Cripps, P.J., Jones, A. and Waterman-Pearson, A.E. (1998) Efficacy and kinetics of carprofen, adminstered preoperatively or postoperatively, for the prevention of pain in dogs undergoing ovariohysterectomy. *Veterinary Surgery* (in press).

Liles, J.H. and Flecknell, P.A. (1992a) The effects of buprenorphine, nalbuphine and butorphanol alone or following halothane anaesthesia on food and water consumption and locomotor movement in rats. *Laboratory Animals* **26**: 180–189.

Liles, J.H. and Flecknell, P.A. (1992b) The use of non-steroidal anti-inflammatory drugs for the relief of pain in laboratory rodents and rabbits. *Laboratory Animals* **26**: 241–255.

Liles, J.H. and Flecknell, P.A. (1993a) A comparison of the effects of buprenorphine, carprofen and flunixin following laparotomy in rats. *Journal of Veterinary Pharmacology and Therapeutics* **17**: 284–290.

Liles, J.H. and Flecknell, P.A. (1993b) The effects of surgical stimulus on the rat and the influence of analgesic treatment. *British Veterinary Journal* **149**: 515–525.

Liles, J.H., Flecknell, P.A., Roughan, J.A. and Cruz-Madorran, I. (1997) Influence of oral buprenorphine, oral naltrexone or morphine on the effects of laparotomy in the rat. *Laboratory Animal* **32**: 149–161.

Lowe, J.E. and Hilfiger, J. (1986) Analagesic and sedative effects of detomidine compared to xylazine in a colic model using IV and IM routes of administration. *Acta Veterinaria Scandinavica* **82** (Suppl): 85–95.

Machin, K.L. (1999) Amphibian pain and analgesia. *Journal of Zoo and Wildlife Medicine* **30**: 2–10.

Martin, A.R. and Wickelgren, W.O. (1971) Sensory cells in the spinal cord of the sea lamprey. *Journal of Physiology* **212**: 65–83.

McCarthy, R.N., Jeffcott, L.B. and Clarke, I.J. (1993) Preliminary studies on the use of plasma beta endorphin in horses as an indicator of stress and pain. *Journal of Equine Veterinary Science* **13**: 216–219.

McGeown, D., Danbury, T.C., Waterman-Pearson, A.E. and Kestin, S.C. (1999) Effect of carprofen on lameness in broiler chickens. *Veterinary Record* **144**: 668–671.

McGlone, J.J. and Hellman, J.M. (1988) Local and general anesthetic effects on behaviour and performance of two- and seven-week old castrated and uncastrated piglets. *Journal of Animal Science* **66**: 3049–3058.

McGrath, P. (1990) Pain assessment in children – a practical approach. *Advances in Pain Research and Therapy* **15**: 5–30.

McGrath, P.J. and Unruh, A.M. (1989) *Pain in Children and Adolescents*. Elsevier, Amsterdam.

McIlvaine, W., Knox, R.K., Fennessey, P.V. and Goldstein, M. (1988) Continuous infusion of bupivacaine via intrapleural catheter for analgesia after thoracotomy in children. *Anesthesiology* **69**: 261–264.

Mellor, D. and Stafford, K. (1999) Assessing and minimising the distress caused by painful husbandry procedures in ruminants. *In Practice* **21**: 436–446.

Morton, D.B. and Griffiths, P.H.M. (1985) Guidelines on the recognition of pain, distress and discomfort in experimental animals and an hypothesis for assessment. *Veterinary Record* **116**: 431–436.

Murrin, K.R. and Rosen, M. (1985) Pain measurement. In: Smith, G. and Covino, B.G. (eds) *Acute Pain*. Butterworths, London, pp 104–132.

Nolan, A., Livingston, A. and Waterman, A.E. (1987) Investigation of the antinociceptive activity of buprenorphine in sheep. *British Journal of Pharmacology* **92**: 527–533.

Nolan, A., Waterman, A.E. and Livingston, A. (1988) The correlation of the thermal and mechanical antinociceptive activity of pethidine hydrochloride with plasma concentrations of the drug in sheep. *Journal of Veterinary Pharmacology and Therapeutics* **11**: 94–102.

Paul-Murphy, J. (1998) Addressing pain in the avian patient. *Proceedings of the American Association of Zoological Veterinarians and American Association of Wildife Veterinarians Joint Conference*, pp 466–469.

Pert, C.B., Aposhian, D. and Snyder, S.H. (1974) Phylogenetic distribution of opiate receptor binding. *Brain Research* **75**: 356–371.

Raekallio, M., Taylor, P.M. and Bloomfield, M. (1997a) A comparison of methods for evaluation of pain and distress after orthopaedic surgery in horses. *Journal of Veterinary Anaesthesia* **24**: 17–20.

Raekallio, M., Taylor, P.M. and Bennett, R.C. (1997b) Preliminary investigations of pain and analgesia assessment in horses given phenylbutazone or placebo after arthroscopic surgery. *Veterinary Surgery* **26**: 150–155.

Rosenblum, P.M. and Peter, R.E. (1989) Evidence for the involvement of endogenous opioids in the regulation of gonadotropin secretion in male goldfish, *Carassius auratus*. *General and Comparative Endocrinology* **73**: 21–27.

Roughan, J. and Flecknell, P.A. (1997) Effects of surgery and analgesic administration on exploratory behaviour in the rat. *Proceedings of the Sixth Federation of European Laboratory Animal Science Associations symposium*. RSM Press, London, pp 30–32.

Sawyer, D. and Rech, R.H. (1987) Analgesia and behavioral effects of butorphanol, nalbuphine, and pentazocine in the cat. *Journal of the American Animal Hospital Association* **23**: 438–446.

Sawyer, D., Rech, R.H., Durham, R.A., Adams, T., Richter, M.A. and Striler, E.L. (1991) Dose response to butorphanol administered subcutaneously to increase visceral nociceptive threshold in dogs. *American Journal of Veterinary Research* **52**: 1826–1830.

Sawyer, D.C., Rech, R.H., Adams, T., Durham, R.A., Richter, M.A. and Striler, E.L. (1992) Analgesia and behavioral responses of dogs given oxymorphone-acepromazine and meperidine-acepromazine after methoxyflurane and halothane anesthesia. *American Journal of Veterinary Research* 53(**8**): 1361–1368.

Schatzmann, U., Gugelmann, M., Von Cranach, J., Ludwig, B.M. and Rehm, W.F. (1990) Pharmacodynamic evaluation of the peripheral pain inhibition by carprofen and flunixin in the horse. *Schweizer Archive für Tierheilkunde* 132(**9**): 497–504.

Schatzmann, U., Weishaupt, M.A. and Straub, R. (1994) Pain models in the horse: quantification of lameness by accelerometric measurements. *Journal of Veterinary Anaesthesia* **21**: 42.

Scott, J., Huskissen, E.C. (1976) Graphic representation of pain. Pain **2**: 175–184.

Silver, I.A., Brown, P.N., Goodship, A.E., et al (1983) A clinical and experimental study of tendon injury, healing and treatment in the horse. *Equine Veterinary Journal* **1** (Suppl): 23–35.

Slingsby, L.S. and Waterman-Pearson, A.E. (1998) Comparison of pethidine, buprenorphine and ketoprofen for postoperative analgesia after ovariohysterectomy in the cat. *Veterinary Record* **143**: 185–189.

Smith, J.A. and Boyd, K.M. (eds) (1991) *Lives in the Balance.* Oxford University Press, Oxford.

Stevens, C.W. (1992) Mini-review – alternatives to the use of mammals for pain research. *Life Sciences* **50**: 901–912.

Stevens, C.W. and Kirkendall, K. (1992) Time course and magnitude of tolerance to the analgesic effects of systemic morphine in amphibians. *Life Sciences* **52**: 111–116.

Stevens, C.W. and Roth, K.S. (1997) Supra-spinal administration of opioids with selectivity for mu, delta and kappa opioid receptors produces analgesia in amphibians. *European Journal of of Pharmacology* **331**: 15–21.

Stevens, C.W., Klopp, A.J. and Facello, J.A. (1994) Analgesic potency of mu and kappa opioids after systemic administration in amphibians 1. *Journal of Pharmacology and Experimental Therapeutics* 269(**3**): 1086–1093.

Stoskopf, M.K. (1994) Analgesia in birds, amphibians and fish. *Investigative Ophthalmology and Visual Science* **35**: 775–780.

Taber, R.I. (1974) Predictive value of analgesic assays in mice and rats. *Advances in Biochemical Psychopharmacology* **8**: 191–221.

Thornton, P.D. and Waterman-Pearson, A.E. (1999) Quantification of the pain and distress responses to castration in young lambs. *Research in Veterinary Science* **66**: 107–118.

Welsh, E.M., Gettinby, G. and Nolan, A.M. (1993) Comparison of a visual analogue scale and a numerical rating scale for assessment of lameness, using sheep as a model. *American Journal of Veterinary Research* 54(**6**, June): 976–983.

Wood, G.N., Molony, V. and Fleetwood-Walker, S.M. (1991) Effects of local anaesthesia and intravenous naloxone on the changes in behaviour and plasma concentrations of cortisol produced by castration and tail docking with tight rubber rings in young lambs. *Research in Veterinary Science* **51**: 193–199.

Wright, E.M., Marcella, K.L. and Woodson, J.F. (1985) Animal pain: evaluation and control. *Laboratory Animals* **14**: 20–30.

MANAGEMENT OF POSTOPERATIVE AND OTHER ACUTE PAIN

5

P. Dobromylskyj, P.A. Flecknell, B.D. Lascelles, P.J. Pascoe,
P. Taylor, A. Waterman-Pearson

Acute pain can occur following elective surgical procedures, trauma and a wide range of medical conditions, particularly those associated with a marked inflammatory component, such as otitis externa and pancreatitis (see chapter 3). As discussed earlier, this pain should be prevented or alleviated, and a range of different analgesic agents are available that can be used safely and effectively in animals (see chapter 3). When formulating an analgesic regimen for a particular patient, several factors need to be considered:

- What is the likely severity of pain, and what is its anticipated duration?
- Which drug or drugs should be administered, and at what doses?
- Are there any special factors that will influence the choice of analgesic, e.g. the species of animal, any pre-existing medical condition, or any particular features of the current condition and the type of pain?
- What facilities are available for management of the patient? Will the patient be hospitalised, or treated as an out-patient? What level of nursing care and monitoring of the animal is available? Are there facilities for continuous infusion of analgesics?

It is also helpful to draw a distinction between pain associated with elective surgical procedures, and pain following trauma or other conditions. Pain following elective surgery can largely be prevented by the use of analgesics before surgery is undertaken – a technique termed 'pre-emptive analgesia' – combined with postoperative top-ups, whereas established pain can only be controlled. Experience in man, coupled with research studies in animals, suggests that effective control of established pain is more difficult to achieve than prevention of pain by early use of analgesics. When using pre-emptive analgesic techniques, use of a single class of analgesic, even at high doses, may not be sufficient to control pain. In situations where severe pain has already been experienced, e.g. after major accidental trauma, pain control using a single analgesic will be even more difficult. In many circumstances, it is preferable to use two or more different analgesics, so-called 'multimodal pain therapy', to provide the most effective pain relief. These concepts are discussed in more detail below, followed by a summary of the particular considerations in different animal species. This chapter concludes with a series of recommendations for controlling pain in a range of different clinical conditions, to provide some initial assistance for formulating pain management strategies. The problems that arise when managing certain clinical problems, e.g. the trauma patient, and those with impaired organ function, are discussed in chapter 6.

Timing of analgesic administration

One of the most important advances in the control of perioperative pain has been the realisation that the timing of analgesic intervention may have a significant bearing on the intensity of postoperative pain. The concept was originally formulated early in the 20th century by Crile (Crile 1913) based on clinical observations. Crile suggested the use of regional blocks with local anaesthetics, in conjunction with general anaesthesia, to prevent postoperative pain in humans and also the formation of painful scars caused by alterations in the central nervous system as a result of the noxious stimulation caused during surgery. Interest in this concept was revived when it was found that changes in the central processing of noxious stimuli occurred in response to peripheral injury (Coderre et al 1993, Richmond et al 1993). This change was suppressed to a greater extent by administration of opioids before, rather than after, injury (Woolf & Wall 1986, Dickenson & Sullivan 1987, Chapman & Dickenson 1994). These initial findings led to the development of the concept of 'pre-emptive analgesia' – administration of analgesics before noxious stimulation begins, to prevent the adverse central nervous system (CNS) changes that this stimulation induces. The physiological changes that produce this central hypersensitivity, and result in more severe pain, are discussed in more detail in chapter 2. To be most effective, pre-emptive analgesia must prevent the noxious information from reaching the central nervous system. It should also aim to reduce or eliminate peripheral inflammation, which in itself augments input into the CNS, so aggravating central hypersensitivity.

A positive effect of pre-emptive drug administration has been found experimentally (Woolf and Wall 1986, Dickenson & Sullivan 1987, Lascelles et al 1995) and clinically in animals given opioids (Lascelles et al 1997) and NSAIDs (Welsh et al 1997, Lascelles et al, 1998). To gain maximum benefit, the matching of nociceptive input and analgesic medication is crucial to exploiting the clinical benefit of pre-emptive analgesia. In other words, the greater the surgical stimulus expected, the greater the degree of pre-emptive analgesia that must be administered. It is also important to appreciate that a single dose of analgesic, administered prior to surgery, will not usually be all the analgesia that will be required. Additional analgesic medication will still be needed in the postoperative period, but this pain will be more easily controlled because pre-emptive analgesia has been used. A further practical advantage of pre-emptive analgesia is that it will often reduce the dose of anaesthetic drugs required, and by integrating analgesic therapy into a balanced anaesthetic regimen, patient safety can be improved, in addition to providing more effective pain relief (see below).

Animals which are presented for treatment that already have established pain, e.g. following a road traffic accident, will not have had analgesics administered prior to the trauma. Nevertheless, administering analgesics as soon as is practicable is still of significant benefit. The longer pain is established, the greater will be the degree of central hypersensitivity, and the more difficult pain management becomes. Of particular interest in this respect is the effect of ketamine, as this drug has the potential to reverse central hypersensitivity because of its actions as an NMDA antagonist (see chapter 3) (Tverskoy et al 1994). Administration of ketamine at subanaesthetic doses (e.g. 0.1 mg/kg in dogs and cats) may help provide analgesia in such cases, although no clinical trials have been carried out to confirm the practical significance of this effect. However, recent studies in dogs and cats have shown that perioperative ketamine reduces postoperative pain scores up to 18 hours later (Slingsby 1999)

'Multimodal' pain therapy

Clinical pain arises from a combination of central and peripheral hypersensitivity involving a multiplicity of pathways, mechanisms and transmitter systems, so it is unlikely that a single class of analgesic will completely alleviate pain, irrespective of the dose used. In order to provide completely effective clinical pain relief, drugs of different classes will be required, each acting on different parts of the pain system. This concept is quite easy to apply in clinical practice, e.g. by combining the use of opioids with NSAIDs. The opioid acts centrally to limit the input of nociceptive information into the CNS and so reduces central hypersensitivity. In contrast, the NSAID acts peripherally to decrease inflammation during and after surgery, and thus limit the nociceptive information entering the CNS as a result of the inflammation, and also acts centrally to limit the central changes induced by the nociceptive information that does get through. By acting on different points of the pain pathways, the combination is more effective than either drug given alone. Adding a local anaesthetic to this regimen can provide additional analgesia by blocking specific nerve pathways, and so further improve the degree of pain control (Fig. 5.1).

Using combinations of different classes of analgesics can also overcome some of the problems associated with differences in the speed of onset of action of the various agents. In a study comparing the degree of postoperative analgesia provided by pethidine and carprofen in dogs, animals which received pethidine had good analgesia immediately following recovery from anaesthesia, compared to animals which received carprofen (Lascelles et al 1994). In contrast, dogs receiving carprofen had better analgesia later in the post-surgical period. Similar results were seen in cats (Slingsby & Waterman-Pearson 1996). Clearly, combining the two analgesics would provide a more effective regimen for controlling postoperative pain than either used alone.

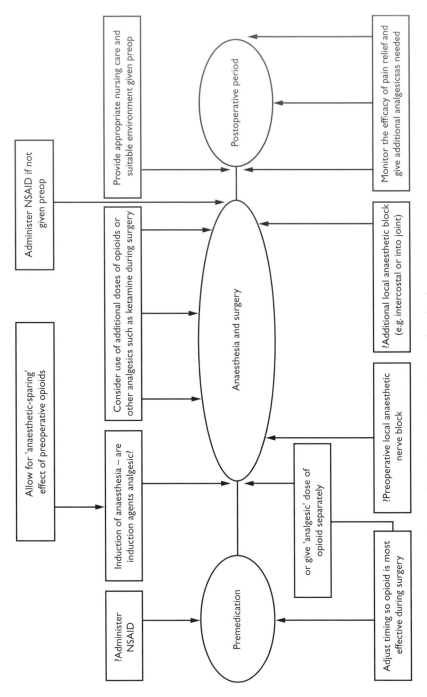

Figure 5.1 Some of the perioperative considerations regarding the use of analgesics.

Anaesthesia and analgesia

Anaesthesia does not necessarily equate with analgesia. General anaesthesia produces loss of consciousness, so the animal cannot perceive pain, but in unconscious animals, noxious stimuli will still be transmitted to and processed by the CNS. Although these noxious stimuli will not be perceived consciously as pain, central hypersensitivity can still develop in the spinal cord and brain, and so postoperative pain perception will be heightened. Some anaesthetic agents do have analgesic effects (e.g. ketamine and alpha-2 adrenoreceptor agonists) and analgesics may be used as part of the anaesthetic regimen (e.g. opioids).

Perioperative analgesic protocols

One way to design an analgesic protocol is outlined below. The three main points to bear in mind are:

- Use analgesics as early as possible – beginning preoperatively
- Use more than one class of analgesic agent, acting at different points on the pain pathways
- Match the doses and duration of action of the analgesics to the degree of expected trauma from surgery.

Once the anaesthetic protocol has been decided, consideration should be given to which analgesics are required. Two practical examples illustrate this: both regimens could be used for ovariohysterectomy in the cat, but the analgesic regimen required is likely to differ.

Protocol 1: *Preanaesthetic medication with acepromazine, followed by induction of anaesthesia with thiopentone and maintenance with halothane.*

Neither acepromazine, thiopentone nor halothane provide any analgesia, so consider giving an opioid, e.g. pethidine (meperidine), as premedication. Pethidine and other opioids have a sedative or calming effect in cats, particularly when combined with a phenothiazine like acepromazine. However, the doses used in combination with acepromazine (e.g. 3–5 mg/kg pethidine) for sedation may be too low to provide significant analgesia, and it may be preferable to use a higher dose of pethidine (5–10 mg/kg i.m.) alone to provide both sedation and analgesia. If an opioid is used preoperatively, sufficient time must be allowed for it to act effectively. Pethidine has a short onset of action (approximately 5 min), but if buprenorphine were selected, a longer delay (30–40 min) would be required before commencing anaesthesia and surgery. Pethidine has a short duration of action in normal animals (90–120 min) although its action is prolonged following anaesthesia, as metabolism is reduced. Thus, pethidine would provide sufficient analgesia intraoperatively for such a relatively brief surgical procedure, but would not provide prolonged postoperative analgesia. Either additional pethidine could be administered postoperatively, or an NSAID such as carprofen, ketoprofen or meloxicam could be incorporated into the analgesic protocol. If carprofen is used, it can also be administered preoperatively, to have an additional 'pre-emptive' effect. Administering pethidine would enable the dose of thiopentone used for induction to be reduced (by 50% or more) and it would also lower the concentration of halothane required for maintenance of anaesthesia (by 0.5–1%).

Protocol 2: *Induction and maintenance of anaesthesia with a combination of ketamine and medetomidine.*

This regimen will provide very good intraoperative analgesia, and the use of ketamine may further help prevent central sensitisation (Slingsby & Waterman-Pearson 1998). Postoperatively, however, additional analgesia is likely to be needed, especially if the medetomidine is reversed with atipamezole. Administration of a potent NSAID, preferably preoperatively, may be sufficient.

In both examples, it would be important to assess the animal regularly postoperatively to ensure the analgesic regimen was adequate. There are many other anaesthetic and analgesic regimens that could be used in these circumstances. The choice will be influenced by many factors, including the preferences and experience of the anaesthetist, but the regimens should be evaluated critically in the light of the general principles outlined earlier.

If, in contrast to a moderate procedure such as ovariohysterectomy, more traumatic surgery was planned, then the use of pure μ agonists, at relatively high doses, will be needed to provide effective pain relief. Morphine or oxymorphone, rather than pethidine, might be preferable, as they have a greater maximal analgesic effect, and longer duration of action. In practical terms, however, these agents may not be readily available. A recent survey of UK practices has shown that the pure μ agonists are not widely available (Capner et al 1999), and a similar situation is likely to exist in much of the rest of Europe. Partial μ agonists such as buprenorphine can be used, and when given at relatively high dose rates (e.g. 40 μg/kg in cats, 20 μg/kg in dogs) good analgesia can be produced. There is probably little clinical significance to the 'bell-shaped' dose – response curve reported for these agents (Cowan et al 1977), and more recent reports have shown high doses to simply produce longer periods of analgesia (Dum & Herz 1981).

Both partial agonists and mixed agonist–antagonists, such as butorphanol, do show a plateau effect, so once a certain degree of analgesia has been produced, increasing the dose rate does not improve the degree of analgesia. This can be a limiting factor when using these drugs to control severe pain. In these circumstances, a μ agonist (such as morphine) may be required. If buprenorphine or butorphanol has been administered, but has not fully controlled the animal's pain, it may antagonise the effects of a subsequent dose of morphine. Although this would be expected from the pharmacology of the agents, in practical terms administration of morphine or oxymorphone in these circumstances *does* usually produce an increased analgesic effect. Paradoxically, buprenorphine or butor-phanol can be used to good effect postoperatively to reverse the μ opioid com-ponent of a balanced anaesthetic regimen (see below), whilst maintaining an analgesic effect.

With the exception of buprenorphine and methadone, the opioids available for clinical use in animals have relatively short (<4h) duration of action. This can lead to a failure to provide analgesia continuously, particularly overnight. To overcome this problem, analgesics can be administered by continuous infusion. This technique is well established in man, and has been shown to be very effect-ive in controlling pain. Infusions of analgesics have the advantage of maintaining effective plasma levels of the analgesic, so providing continuous pain relief. This is in contrast to intermittent injections, where pain may return before the next dose of analgesic is administered (Fig. 5.2). This technique can pose some practi-cal problems in animals, but is no more difficult than maintaining intravenous fluid therapy. In larger species (>3–4kg body weight), a lightweight infusion pump can be bandaged directly to the animal and continuous infusion made simply by means of a butterfly type needle anchored subcutaneously or intra-muscularly. Alternatively, the infusion pump can be attached via an extension tube directly to an intravenous catheter. Although it is possible to add analgesics to a burette on a fluid administration set, this is potentially hazardous – if the rate of fluid administration increases because of failure of the drip controller, overdose could occur. When analgesics are to be administered by continuous infusion, the infusion rate can be calculated from a knowledge of the pharmaco-kinetics of the analgesic to be used – the volume of distribution (the theoretical space in the body available to contain the drug) and its rate constants (Mather 1983, Flecknell 1996). If these data are not readily available, an approximation that appears successful in clinical use is as follows: calculate the total dose

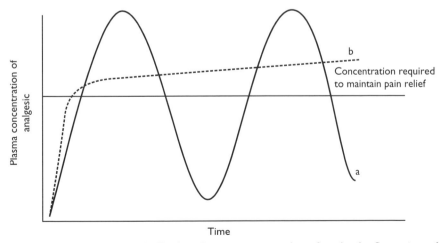

Figure 5.2 Maintenance of effective plasma concentration of analgesic. Comparison of continuous infusion (a) and intermittent administration (b) of drug.

required over the period of infusion, reduce this by half and set the pump infusion rate accordingly; administer a single, normal dose of the drug as an initial loading dose and start the infusion. The rate can then be adjusted depending upon the animal's responses.

NSAIDs are frequently considered for use in a perioperative analgesic protocol. If possible, they should be administered preoperatively. This is not without risk, as NSAIDs that are potent inhibitors of cyclooxygenase (e.g. flunixin and ketoprofen) can occasionally precipitate acute renal failure, most notably in the dog and cat. If, during anaesthesia, there is a degree of relative or absolute hypovolaemia, or if there is hypotension, locally produced prostaglandins help maintain renal blood flow (see chapter 3). Administration of a potent cyclooxygenase inhibitor can remove the protective effects of these prostaglandins, and leave the kidney vulnerable to damage. In these situations, the choice of a prostaglandin-sparing NSAID is preferable. At the time of writing, the only NSAID of this type available for veterinary clinical use is carprofen, and this drug is licensed in several countries for preoperative administration in the dog and cat. However, it is possible that other NSAIDs could also be administered safely preoperatively, and additional information is likely to become available as clinical trials are completed. Horses do not appear to be as vulnerable as dogs and cats to the adverse effects of NSAIDs on renal autoregulation and NSAIDs are frequently administered prior to surgery in this species. Information concerning the susceptibility of other species is very limited, although NSAIDs are often used pre- and intraoperatively in cattle without clinically apparent problems (Taylor, personal communication). If NSAIDs are not administered preoperatively, they should be administered during recovery unless contraindicated for other reasons.

Local anaesthetics can be a valuable adjunct to analgesic protocols. Local infiltration of the surgical site, either before or following surgery, or use of regional or epidural blockade provides another mode of analgesia (see below). Although not directly relevant to postoperative analgesia, it is worth noting that use of topical preparations, e.g. lidocaine and prilocaine (EMLA cream, Astra), can provide pain-free venepuncture. This can be particularly useful in excitable or fractious animals. These local anaesthetic creams provide full-skin thickness analgesia. The skin should be shaved, the cream applied quite thickly in a layer approximately 2–3 mm thick, and covered with a waterproof dressing. Some commercial products are supplied with an adhesive plastic bandage, but plastic food wrapper (e.g. clingfilm) can be used. The plastic bandage is then covered with an adhesive dressing to prevent the animal interfering with the cream. After 30–60 minutes (depending upon skin thickness), the dressing is removed and the skin wiped clean, and venepuncture carried out (Flecknell et al 1990a). The technique is particularly useful when placing large-diameter catheters for fluid therapy.

Preanaesthetic administration of analgesics often enables the dose of other anaesthetic agents to be reduced. This should always be considered when planning the overall protocol, to avoid inadvertent anaesthetic overdosage. Provided this effect is recognised, it is usually regarded as beneficial, since the undesirable effects of agents such as halothane (e.g. hypotension) are dose-dependent, so that reducing the concentration needed for maintenance will increase patient safety.

Use of mixed agonist/antagonists to reverse anaesthesia

If a pure μ agonist is used as a major component of an anaesthetic regimen, e.g. when using neuroleptanalgesic mixtures such as fentanyl/fluanisone (Hypnorm, Janssen) or fentanyl/droperidol (Innovar Vet, Mallinckrodt), excellent intraoperative pain relief is provided. This will extend into the postoperative period, even when short-acting analgesics such as fentanyl are used, because of the high dose rates administered (Flecknell et al 1989). A disadvantage of this may be that the regimen produces significant respiratory depression, coupled with prolonged sedation, and reversal of the μ opioid may be considered desirable. If a μ antagonist, such as naloxone, is used, then this will reverse the sedation and respiratory depression, but will also either completely reverse, or markedly reduce the analgesic effect of the μ agonist (e.g. fentanyl). This can be avoided by using a mixed agonist/antagonist, such as butorphanol, or even a partial agonist such as buprenorphine. In these circumstances, the effects of the fentanyl (or other μ agonist) are reversed, but continued analgesia is provided (Flecknell et al 1989). This effect has been demonstrated in man, following the use of high dose morphine or fentanyl (de Castro & Viars 1968, Latasch et al 1984); in the dog, after the use of oxymorphone and alfentanil (Flecknell et al 1990b, McCrackin et al 1994); and in rabbits and small rodents after the use of fentanyl (Hu et al 1992). As neuroleptanalgesic regimens are particularly popular in rabbits and small rodents, the technique is of most practical value in these species. It can, however, also be used effectively in larger animals.

Local anaesthetic and analgesic techniques

Local anaesthetic techniques block action potential transmission in all nerve fibres, including those transmitting nociceptive information. They are therefore ideal for providing pre-emptive analgesia, as they can block all nociceptive input. Because of the complete sensory block that is provided, they markedly decrease the requirement for general anaesthetic agents. Local anaesthetic techniques are relatively easy to implement, even in small mammals.

Topical

Local anaesthetic can be deposited around exposed nerves during surgery, e.g. during forelimb amputations the nerves of the brachial plexus should be bathed in local anaesthetic for 2–3 minutes prior to transection (approximately 5 ml of 0.5% bupivacaine is used in a 20 kg dog). Alternatively, the local anaesthetic can be injected directly into the perineurium of the nerves that are being sectioned. Although surgery will have commenced, the additional nociceptive input following sectioning of the nerves is considerable, and prior blockade will have a significant effect in decreasing postoperative pain and possibly reduces the chance of phantom limb pain developing.

Local anaesthetic can be sprayed on exposed nasal turbinate mucosa following nasal surgery, and local anaesthetic gels can be spread on the rectum following rectal or perirectal surgery to provide analgesia and decrease tenesmus. Topical local anaesthetic can also be used to good effect during major aural surgery and for extraocular eye surgery (Ophthaine, Squibb).

Local infiltration

Local anaesthetic infiltrated around the surgical site can also provide sufficient analgesia to allow suturing or minor surgery in conscious animals. The stinging sensation associated with lidocaine infiltration can be significantly reduced by mixing with sodium bicarbonate (1 part of $1\,mol/L$ $NaHCO_3$ with 9 parts of 1 or 2% lidocaine mixed immediately prior to injection). Discomfort is also reduced by warming the local anaesthetic to body temperature prior to injection (there is no need to store local anaesthetics in a refrigerator). When infiltrating local anaesthetic into a surgical site after more major surgery, carried out under general anaesthesia, care should be taken to infiltrate each of the tissue planes, so that effective analgesia is provided. Infiltration of local anaesthetic into surgical wounds does not delay healing significantly.

Regional blockade

Local anaesthetics can be infiltrated along a line to block all of the nerves supplying a region. For example, local anaesthetic can be injected around a distal limb or around the base of a digit prior to distal surgery or amputation, respectively. A detailed knowledge of the anatomy of the area is not required. When blocking extremities with such 'ring blocks', local anaesthetics without adrenaline should be used to prevent tissue ischaemia caused by the vasoconstrictive effects of adrenaline on local blood vessels. Regional blocks are frequently used in farm animal species: for example the inverted-L block used in cattle to block the paravertebral nerves supplying the abdominal wall. However, if excessive volumes of local anaesthetic are used, toxicity can result; care is especially needed in small patients.

Intravenous regional anaesthesia

Local anaesthetics can be administered into a distal vein of a limb with a tourniquet applied proximally in order to produce analgesia of the area below the tourniquet, prior to carrying out digit amputation or other distal limb surgery in a wide variety of species.

Specific nerve blocks

If the anatomy of the area is known, local anaesthetic can be injected accurately to block the sensory nerves supplying the surgical site. Examples include intercostal nerve blocks following thoracotomy, maxillary and mandibular alveolar nerve blocks, brachial plexus block in small animals, pudendal and paravertebral nerve blocks in cattle and individual nerve blocks to the distal limb in horses. The techniques are reasonably straightforward and are best performed prior to surgery.

Intercostal nerve blocks

An intercostal nerve block abolishes nociceptor input from tissues innervated by the intercostal nerves and can provide very effective analgesia following thoracotomy (Pascoe and Dyson 1993). The procedure does not seem to be associated with impaired ventilation (Gilroy 1982). Due to overlap of innervation, nerves cranial and caudal to the site of the incision must be blocked. The intercostal nerves descend in the intercostal space along the caudal border of each rib, associated with the ventral branches of the intercostal artery and vein. Ideally, the block is performed as high up (dorsally) as possible, near the intervertebral foramen. The needle is advanced onto the rib, and then 'walked' caudally until it enters the tissues behind the caudal border of the rib. After the syringe is aspirated to check that a blood vessel has not been entered, local anaesthetic is injected. This is repeated in order to block three intercostal nerves in front of the incision and three caudal to it, in addition to the site of the incision. A total dose of 1.5 mg/kg of 0.5% bupivacaine is used in dogs, which approximates to 0.5 ml/site in dogs of less than 10 kg, and 1 ml per site in dogs greater than 10 kg. This procedure is best carried out before surgery, after the induction of anaesthesia, to maximise the beneficial effect of the local anaesthetic. Occasionally, a blood vessel may be damaged during injection, and some blood may be present in the chest on thoracotomy. Some surgeons may be concerned about this, and prefer that the block is performed after the completion of surgery. In these circumstances, the local anaesthetic can be injected from the pleural side of the chest wall if desired. This approach also makes location of the nerve and accurate placement of local anaesthetic easier, and also enables blockade of the dorsal branch of the intercostal nerve, by injecting close to the point at which the nerve exits the spinal canal.

Maxillary and mandibular nerve blocks

The maxillary or the mandibular nerve can be blocked as they exit from the infraorbital and mental foramen respectively, to provide analgesia following maxillary and mandibular surgery. Both nerves can be palpated through the skin, and a narrow gauge needle placed in the tissues beside the nerve (e.g. 23–25 G, >1″ length for a dog). Following aspiration to check a vessel has not been entered, 0.5–1.0 ml of bupivacaine (0.5%) is deposited at the site. Again, this procedure is best carried out before surgery, and blocks can be repeated following surgery as necessary; however, conscious animals often resent the injections.

Analgesia is produced over an area extending rostrally from the point of the nerve block. If a larger area of block is required, the needle can be inserted into the infraorbital or mental foramen, and the local anaesthetic deposited further back along the course of the nerve.

Paravertebral nerve block

Paravertebral analgesia was first described by Farquharson (1940) as a means of providing complete and uniform desensitisation of the abdominal wall and peritoneum in order to allow abdominal surgery in the standing cow. Although it is primarily an anaesthetic technique, judicious use of longer-acting local anaesthetic agents can usefully contribute to providing postoperative analgesia following surgery. Clinically, it is certainly easy to detect when the block wears off following laparotomy as cows invariably become duller and show signs of discomfort, which is ameliorated by NSAID administration.

The technique has been variously modified as a result of studies to determine the course of the spinal nerves, in an effort to improve the efficacy of the procedure. In cattle, sheep and goats the technique is widely accepted as superior to infiltration methods to provide complete desensitisation of the flank and is widely used, although in large cattle it is not reliable. In these species a proximal approach to the last thoracic and first three lumbar spinal nerves is favoured in the UK (Hall & Clark 1991), while a distal approach has been advocated in the USA (Cakala 1961). The former technique requires the use of a specific stout and long paravertebral needle but does minimise the volume of local anaesthetic required. The distal approach obviates the need for a special needle, but larger volumes of local anaesthetic are needed as it is more difficult to position the needle reliably adjacent to the nerves. Both techniques require that both the dorsal and ventral branches of each spinal nerve are desensitised so that not only the skin and subcutis, but also the muscles and peritoneum, are desensitised.

In horses paravertebral analgesia has been documented as a means of providing flank anaesthesia to allow standing surgical interventions (Moon & Suler 1993). The technique is technically much more demanding as the transverse processes are impossible to palpate or even reach in all but the thinnest and smallest horse.

In the dog the technique has been described by Michelletto (cited by Hall & Clark 1991) as a way of providing analgesia and good muscle relaxation without respiratory muscle paralysis. There is much to commend in this concept; however, as seven nerves need to be blocked each side, it is a time-consuming exercise to undertake and is not therefore widely performed.

Instillation into a cavity

Local anaesthetic can be flushed into the thoracic cavity through a thoracostomy tube (placed at the time of surgery) to provide analgesia following surgery. The patient should be positioned appropriately to ensure that local anaesthetic bathes the incision for the first 20 minutes following infusion (Thompson & Johnson 1991). When bupivacaine is used, 1–2 mg/kg is infused every 4–6 hours (not exceeding 8 mg/kg on day one, and not exceeding 4 mg/kg on subsequent days (Mazoit et al 1988)). Some clinicians have reported that instillation may be painful when carried out in conscious animals, so care should be taken when using this technique. Bupivacaine should not be used following pericardiectomy due to the risk of cardiotoxicity. If a chest drain is placed, then this can be used for the infusion; alternatively a small catheter can be anchored in place or local anaesthetic instilled directly via a needle. Some chest drains are provided with attachments to allow easy anchoring to the chest wall, or they can be secured using a Chinese finger-trap suture pattern (Fig. 5.3).

Instillation of local anaesthetic into the abdomen can be very effective for upper abdominal pain, but is not very effective for general abdominal pain. Bupivacaine (0.5 mg/kg) or lidocaine (1.0 mg/kg) can also be instilled into joints following surgery once the joint has been effectively sealed (Sammarco et al 1996). A common problem is an inability to inject the full dose into the joint,

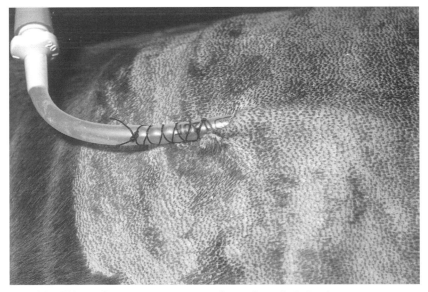

Figure 5.3 Chinese finger-trap suture securing a chest drain in place.

and so the more concentrated solutions of local anaesthetic are generally used. Nevertheless, this technique is extremely simple and provides very effective and safe postoperative analgesia following stifle and shoulder arthrotomies.

Extradural or spinal administration

Local anaesthetics can be administered preoperatively into the extradural ('epidural') or subarachnoid ('spinal') spaces, either alone or in combination with opioids or alpha-2 adrenoreceptor agonists. Spinal (intrathecal) administration of analgesics is rarely used to provide clinical pain relief in animals, but has been used extensively in pain research. Epidural analgesia, using local anaesthetics or other drugs, has extensive clinical applications and is discussed in detail below.

Epidural anaesthesia and analgesia

Indications

Epidural injections can be used to provide anaesthesia of the caudal half of the body or can be used to provide analgesia extending up to the forelimbs. Local anaesthetics can be used at doses that will give total sensory and motor loss to the affected area. This can be useful to provide absolute pain control for surgical procedures or for carrying out postoperative physiotherapy when the movement of the leg is going to be very painful. At lower concentrations, local anaesthetics may be used to provide analgesia without incurring motor deficits but it is difficult to titrate this effect precisely. Even if motor function appears to be relatively normal initially, it is probable that there are some proprioceptive deficits incurred with this approach (Buggy et al 1994). When opioids are used epidurally the expectation is that there will be almost no effect on motor control and that the nociceptive input will be reduced but not totally abolished. Morphine, in particular, can be used to provide a long-lasting analgesic effect from a single injection.

Technique for dogs and cats

1. The site for an epidural injection in both dogs and cats is the lumbosacral space (Fig. 5.4). This can be approached with the animal in lateral or sternal recumbency, but the author (PJP) has had the greatest success with the animal in sternal recumbency with the hind legs extended forward under the body (Fig. 5.5). This position is easy to achieve in the anaesthetised animal but may not be so easy if the animal is awake. (In this case the hind legs can be flexed so the animal is in a normal crouching position.) The lumbosacral space is located by drawing an imaginary line connecting the most dorsally prominent parts of the wings of the ilium; the line should pass through the dorsal spinous process

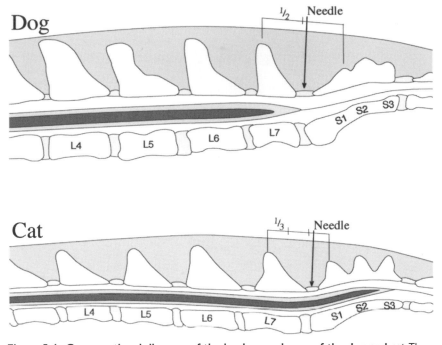

Figure 5.4 Cross-sectional diagram of the lumbosacral area of the dog and cat. The diagram was taken from radiographic images to show the shape of the dorsal spinous processes of the lumbar and sacral vertebrae. Note the difference in the shape of the dorsal spinous process of the first sacral vertebra between the dog and cat. Using L7 and S1 as palpable landmarks the diagram shows that access to the lumbosacral junction is approximately half way between these two points in dogs but is towards the caudal third in cats.

of L7. The most anterior parts of the ilium can also be used as a landmark, and in this case the line joining these two points will normally cross the dorsal spinous process of L6. The lumbosacral space is located immediately posterior to L7 and this can be felt as a depression anterior to the dorsal spinous processes of the sacrum.

2. Once this space has been located, the hair is clipped and the area cleaned as for a routine surgical incision (Fig. 5.6). A spinal needle is used with the size and length depending on the size of the patient:

    <5 kg – 1"×25 G   10–45 kg – 2.5"×22 G
    5–10 kg – 1.5"× 22 G   >45 kg – 3.5"×22 G

3. The operator should put on sterile gloves and use a sterile spinal needle. One hand is used to confirm the landmarks; the needle is positioned over the midline with the bevel of the needle directed rostrally and advanced perpendicular to the skin. It helps to position one's hand so that it is in contact with the animal when penetrating the skin (Fig. 5.7). This contact provides some counterpressure and helps to avoid pushing the needle too far into the animal once the resistance of the skin to penetration has been overcome.

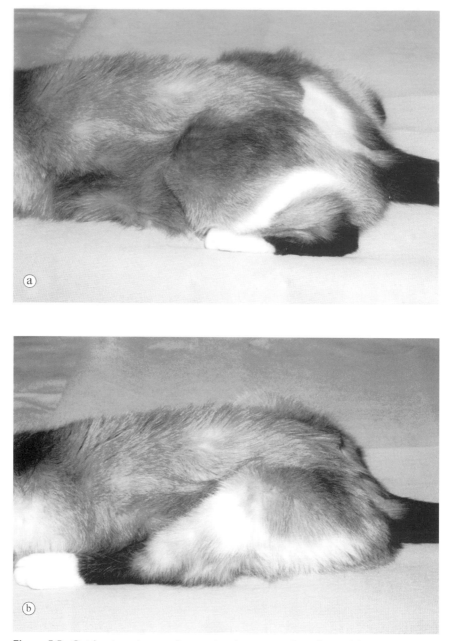

Figure 5.5 Cat in sternal recumbency showing two options for positioning the legs.
(a) With the legs crouched underneath the animal, the external landmarks are often slightly
easier to feel. (b) With the legs extended forward there is an increased tension on the
ligamentum flavum which makes it easier to discern when the ligament has been penetrated.

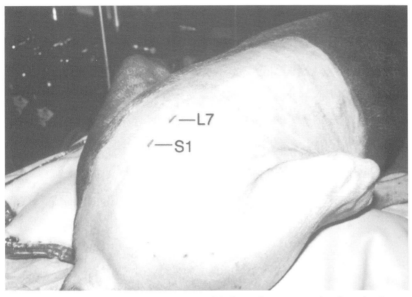

Figure 5.6 Dog in sternal recumbency with lines drawn over the dorsal spinous processes of L7 and S1.

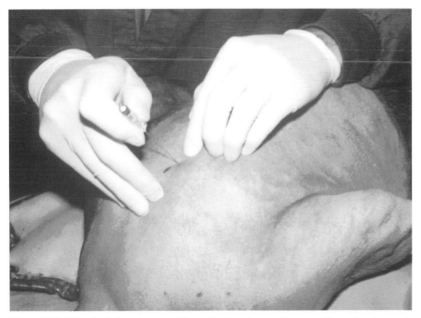

Figure 5.7 Needle being inserted into the lumbosacral space. The index finger of the non-dominant hand is placed on L7 to ensure that the needle is being placed along the midline. The fingers of the dominant hand rest against the dog in order to provide some counterpressure as the needle is inserted through the skin. This helps to prevent the needle from being driven in too deeply once it has gone through the skin.

4. The needle is advanced until it touches bone or penetrates the ligamentum flavum (Figs 5.8 & 5.9). If bone is touched, it is usually the dorsal surface of the vertebral body and this gives an idea of the depth the needle will need to advance to penetrate the ligamentum, which is at the same depth. If the needle encounters bone it should be withdrawn to just below skin level without changing the angle of the needle. Once the needle is at the level of the skin it can be redirected and advanced again. This technique avoids tearing tissue or bending the needle. The needle should only be rotated by 5–10° so that the lumbosacral space is not overshot. When the needle penetrates the ligamentum flavum there is a distinct 'pop'; it should be advanced no further, so that its tip remains just barely beneath the ligament. Most of the blood vessels lie in the ventral part of the spinal canal and one is much less likely to end up with an intravenous penetration if the needle is not pushed in too far. In cats, the spinal cord ends at S1–S2 so it is more likely that the dura will be punctured if the needle is advanced too deeply. At this point one may see the tail twitch, as an indication that the needle has come in contact with the cauda equina.

5. The stylet is removed from the needle and the hub observed for evidence of blood or CSF. If either fluid is seen, then the needle should be withdrawn and repositioned. If CSF is still issuing from the needle, the dose of drug should be reduced to one-quarter of the normal dose. If no fluid is coming out then the following test is carried out: 0.5–1 ml of air is injected and the plunger of the syringe watched carefully. Glass syringes are particularly valuable for this test because the resistance to injection with a glass syringe is much lower than with

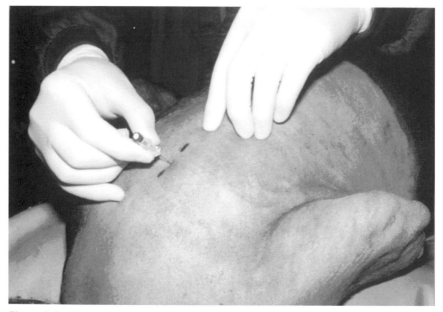

Figure 5.8 The needle has contacted bone and cannot be advanced any further. This is useful because it gives an indication of the depth at which the ligament will be found.

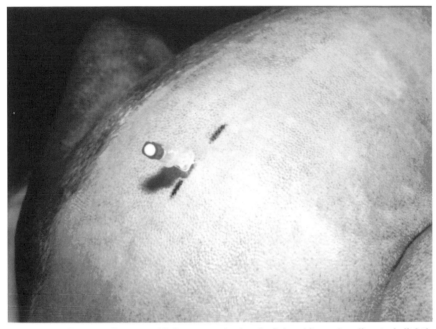

Figure 5.9 **The needle was withdrawn to the level of the skin and redirected slightly more cranially and a 'popping' sensation felt as the needle went through the ligamentum flavum.** Once through the ligament the needle is not advanced any further.

a standard plastic syringe (Fig. 5.10). However, it is quite feasible to use the conventional plastic syringes. The amount of air injected must be limited because excessive amounts in the epidural space will tend to displace a drug from its active site giving rise to a 'patchy' block (Dales et al 1987). If the plunger bounces back at all then the needle is not correctly positioned.

6. Once the test indicates that the needle is correctly placed, the syringe containing the drug is attached and the needle is aspirated first (Fig. 5.11). It is possible for the needle to be in a vein and this would give a loss of resistance to air injection but may not bleed back into the needle because of the negative pressure in the vessel. If blood is aspirated the needle must be removed and replaced. Another technique which helps to ensure accurate placement and maintenance during injection is to allow a small air bubble to be present in the syringe (Fig. 5.12). As the drug is injected this bubble is watched and any evidence of compression means the placement of the needle should be rechecked. The drug injection should be made slowly over about 1–2 minutes (Fig. 5.13). (For doses see Table 5.1.) Lower doses are required in the older patient (the spinal canal is reduced in size due to ageing), the pregnant animal (the spinal canal is reduced in size due to engorgement of the venous sinuses) and the obese animal (the spinal canal is still the same size as the same animal in its lean state). Epidural analgesia with local anaesthetics may block the sympathetic

99

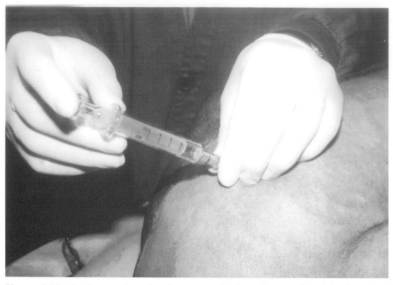

Figure 5.10 A glass syringe has been attached to the needle with about 1 ml of air in it. Note that the non-dominant hand is gripping the needle and resting against the animal in order to prevent the needle from moving in or out. Pressure is being applied to the plunger to test the ease of injection. If a small amount of air is injected and the pressure released on the plunger it will bounce back if the tip of the needle is not in the epidural space.

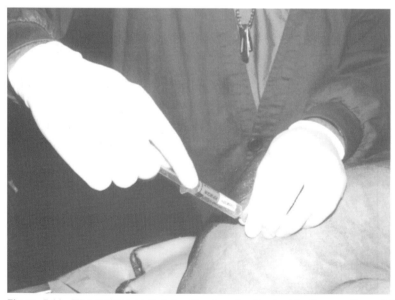

Figure 5.11 The syringe containing the drug is attached to the needle and the plunger pulled back to aspirate from the needle. This is done to ensure that the needle is not in a blood vessel. If blood is aspirated the needle should be removed and another needle used. The needle is still being held firmly to prevent movement.

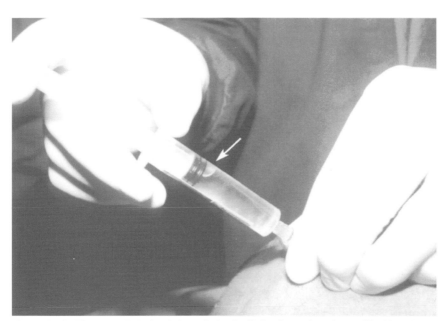

Figure 5.12 The drug is being injected slowly (1–2 minutes) and steadily. Note the small air bubble in the syringe (white arrow). This is a further monitor for the ease of injection. If the needle is dislodged from the epidural space there will be a greater resistance to injection and the air bubble will compress. If this occurs the needle should be replaced into the epidural space and tested again for loss of resistance to injection.

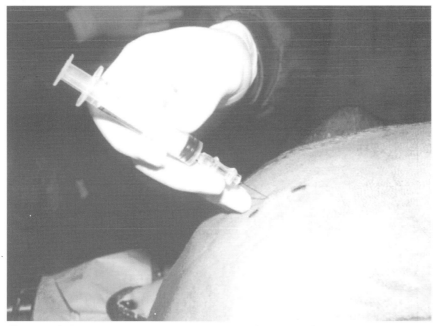

Figure 5.13 The needle and syringe can be withdrawn together.

Drug	Dose	Onset time	Duration
Lidocaine	3–5 mg/kg	5–10 m	1–1.5 h
Lidocaine and epinephrine			
(5 μg/ml)	3–4.5 mg/kg	5–10 m	2–4 h
Mepivacaine	3–4.5 mg/kg	5–10 m	1.5–2 h
Bupivacaine	1–2.5 mg/kg	10–15 m	3–4 h
Morphine	0.1 mg/kg	20–60 m	16–24 h
Meperidine	5–10 mg/kg	5–10 m	1–4 h
Methadone	0.7–1 mg/kg	5–10 m	4–9 h
Oxymorphone	0.05–0.1 mg/kg	20–40 m	7–10 h
Fentanyl	5–10 μg/kg	5–30 m	2–5 h
Sufentanil	0.7–2 μg/kg	5–15 m	4–6 h
Butorphanol	0.25 mg/kg	10–20 m	3 h
Buprenorphine	5–15 μg/kg	60 m	16–24 h
Xylaxine	0.25 mg/kg	5–10 m	1–4 h
Medetomidine	10–15 μg/kg	5–10 m	1–8 h
Morphine and medetomidine	0.1 mg/kg and 1–5 μg/kg		10–16 h
Morphine and bupivacaine	0.1 mg/kg and 1 mg/kg	10–15 m	16–24 h
Morphine infusion	0.3 mg/kg/24 hrs		
Morphine and bupivacaine infusion	0.3 mg/kg/24 hrs and 0.75 mg/kg/24 hrs		

Table 5.1 Dose rates of drugs for epidural use in the dog and cat (see text for dose rates for other species and additional information).

control of blood pressure in the affected area leading to hypotension. This can be treated by loading the animal with fluids (e.g. 20 ml/kg lactated Ringer's) or administering an alpha-1 agonist such as phenylephrine or ephedrine. An epidural injection is contraindicated in patients with any evidence of trauma or infection in the area of the injection, septicaemia or coagulopathies.

Technique for horses

The typical injection site for the horse is between the first and second coccygeal vertebrae (Skarda 1996a). The last sacral and the first coccygeal vertebrae are often fused and the lumbosacral site is a lot more difficult because of the depth of the site (15–20 cm). The intercoccygeal junction is located about 5 cm cranial to the origin of the first tail hairs. The area is shaved and prepared with an antiseptic solution and lidocaine is used to infiltrate the site and the deeper tissues before the final disinfection. The needle (5.0–7.5 cm spinal needle) can then be positioned over the midline in the middle of the intercoccygeal junction and advanced perpendicular to the skin until a 'pop' is felt as the needle penetrates the ligamentum flavum. Alternatively, the needle is placed toward the back of the joint and advanced at about 30° to the horizontal with the idea of sliding the needle along the vertebral canal. In either case a drop of saline placed into the hub of the needle should get drawn into the canal due to the slight negative pressure present in the epidural space ('hanging drop' technique). If this does not happen, the needle placement can be checked using the method described above.

Technique for cattle

The most common epidural injection site in cattle is also the first intercoccygeal junction but it is also feasible to use the sacrococcygeal junction and the lumbosacral junction (Skarda 1996b). The intercoccygeal site is usually located by moving the tail up and down and feeling for the most prominent depression on the midline at the head of the tail. As above, the area is clipped and prepared aseptically and a local anaesthetic injected into the superficial tissue. A 3.5–0.5 cm needle is then used and is applied perpendicular to the skin on the midline. The needle is advanced until it either penetrates the ligamentum flavum or contacts bone. If the latter occurs, the needle should be withdrawn and redirected. Some people advocate advancing the needle to the floor of the canal and then withdrawing a few millimetres in order to have the needle in the centre of the canal. The 'hanging drop' and 'loss of resistance' tests are useful for confirming the placement of the needle.

Locating the lumbosacral space is done by drawing a line across the cranial edges of the tuber sacrale and moving 1–2 cm caudal to that along the midline. The area is clipped and prepared aseptically and the skin and subcutaneous tissues infiltrated with lidocaine. A 15–20 cm needle is needed to attain sufficient depth and is advanced into the intervertebral space perpendicular to the skin. As in other species the needle is advanced until it either penetrates the ligamentum flavum or contacts bone. If the latter occurs, the needle needs to be withdrawn virtually to the skin and redirected cranially or caudally. Tests as described above can be used to confirm the location of the needle. The spinal cord in cattle does not terminate until the sacral region so the needle may penetrate the dura and result in CSF issuing from the needle. Ideally the needle should be removed and a second attempt made but it is acceptable to use a reduced dose of the drug to be injected (about 1/4 of the epidural dose).

Epidural catheterisation

An epidural catheter can be placed using the same landmarks as above, but in order to get the catheter to advance up the epidural canal it is necessary to enter the ligamentum flavum at a shallower angle. Most Tuohy needles will only alter the direction of the catheter by a few degrees and so if the needle is close to perpendicular the catheter seems to bump into the floor of the canal and does not slide easily. To be able to achieve this shallower angle, it is often necessary to make the skin puncture to one side of the first sacral dorsal spinous process and angle the needle towards the midline. In general, it is easier to feel the penetration of the ligament with a Tuohy needle because they are relatively blunt. In order to do this it may be necessary to clip a wider area than one might use for an epidural injection and it is advisable to have a surgical drape over the area so that the catheter does not get contaminated.

Epidural catheters come in a variety of materials and sizes. Most need a 17 or 18 SWG Tuohy or Crawford needle to allow one to pass a 19 or 20 SWG catheter. Some epidural catheters are made of polyamide or a copolymer and come with a wire guide down the middle. Typically, the wire finishes a little before the end of the catheter. Other catheters come with a wire spiral built into the wall of the catheter. These tend to be relatively flexible and have the great advantage that it is almost impossible to kink them and they can remain patent even when tied in a knot! The tip of the catheter may be open or closed (bullet tipped) with multiple side ports. In theory, the bullet-tipped catheter with multiple side ports is less likely to traumatise the tissue and provide more even spread of the injected fluid, but this is not always so (Junega et al 1995). When placing the catheters with a central wire guide it may be necessary to retract the wire a little to keep the tip flexible; however, care must be taken that the catheter does not flip back on itself and kink. In people, the incidence of vascular catheterisation with this catheter was 8%, while this was reduced to 6.7% when a softer polyurethane catheter was used (Rolbin et al 1987). The incidence of venous catheterisation and paresthesias was much lower with the wire-reinforced catheter in people when compared with a copolymer bullet-tip catheter or a polyamide open–tip catheter (Junega et al 1995, 1996). However, because these catheters are more flexible they are more difficult to thread up the canal.

When preparing for epidural catheterisation it is important to check first that the catheter will go through the needle and to get a 'feel' for how much resistance occurs when the catheter reaches the tip of the needle and changes direction. Catheters have centimetre markings which give an indication of the length of the needle and then allow one to measure how much of the catheter has been pushed beyond the end of the needle. It is essential to measure the animal beforehand to determine how much catheter is to be inserted. For a hind leg procedure the catheter may only need to be inserted 2–4 cm but it is a good idea to insert a little more into the epidural space since the catheter will tend to back out when the needle is being removed or the catheter is being fixed to the skin. For an abdominal procedure one may want to insert the catheter up to L2/3, while for a thoracotomy it might be advanced up to T5/6. Occasionally for a foreleg procedure we will advance the catheter up to T1/2. If the catheter has been advanced beyond the end of the needle but cannot be advanced to the desired position no attempt should be made to withdraw the catheter through the needle because it is very easy to shear off the catheter. The needle and catheter must be withdrawn together and then the catheter can be pulled out carefully under direct vision, ensuring that it does not get caught on a sharp edge of the needle.

Once the catheter is in place the needle is removed, taking care not to remove the catheter as well. A Tuohy/Bohrst adapter is then clamped on to the outside end of the catheter and a PRN or bacterial filter and PRN. The catheter is then fixed to the skin at its exit site using a piece of tape as a 'butterfly,' which is then sutured or stapled to the skin. Further tape is applied along the length of the catheter and this is attached to the back of the dog. One can either use a transparent sterile sticky surgery drape or one can do this with strips of Elastoplast (Elasticon), making sure that one has access to the injection site on the catheter. The dog should have an Elizabethan collar placed so that it cannot chew the catheter.

These comments apply to placement of epidural catheters in dogs only because, to date, this author (PJP) has not had success placing epidural catheters in cats in a clinical setting. Even using a 20 SWG Tuohy needle and a 24 SWG blunt-tipped catheter, I have been unable to place it without getting it in a subdural space.

Local anaesthetics

The sites of action of local anaesthetics given epidurally are still somewhat controversial but are thought to be the intradural spinal nerve roots and the periphery of the spinal cord. The final effect of a local anaesthetic in the epidural space is not only related to its lipid solubility but also to properties such as the pK_a, the pH of the solution and that of the tissue, and the protein binding capacity of the drug. The pK_as of the amide local anaesthetics are fairly similar, ranging from 7.92 for mepivacaine to 8.21 for bupivacaine, so the cationic form of the drug predominates slightly at physiological pH, but it is the base form which is required for penetration of the lipid membrane. It is, however, the ionic form which is involved in blocking the sodium channel. The onset of action is partly dependent on lipid solubility and partly on the concentration of the drug. The permeability of lidocaine and bupivacaine is fairly similar despite the differences in their lipid solubility. The onset of action of bupivacaine in dogs is similar to that of lidocaine, of the order of 3–4 minutes until onset of a motor block (Lebeaux 1973), but the time to peak effect is considerably slower with bupivacaine when used clinically (Heath et al 1985). In this latter study the effectiveness of the block was also influenced by the concentration of bupivacaine, with 0.75% giving a slightly higher success rate than 0.5%. The duration of the block appears to be related to the protein binding capacity of the drug, with drugs like lidocaine and mepivacaine which are 65–75% protein bound having a duration of action of 1.5–4.0 hours, while bupivacaine and ropivacaine, which are more highly protein bound (99%), have prolonged effects (3–6 hours) (Feldman et al 1996). The duration of block can also be affected by the addition of an alpha-1 agonist to the local anaesthetic. Epinephrine is the most commonly used drug for this purpose and prolongs the block with lidocaine and mepivacaine but does not appear to do so with bupivacaine or ropivacaine (Feldman & Covino 1988). The addition of epinephrine decreases the vascular uptake of the drugs and thereby reduces the likelihood of systemic toxicity.

Recently there has been renewed interest in using local anaesthetics to provide a sensory block without interfering with motor control. The mechanisms behind this differential blockade are not well understood. Some have suggested that it is a result of the action of the local anaesthetic in the nerve roots, where it is necessary to block a certain number of nodes of Ranvier in myelinated fibres to prevent conduction. In the unmyelinated C fibres even a short length of axonal block will inhibit transmission of a signal. Part of the differential block may be a result of the frequency of discharge – local anaesthetics are taken up more rapidly by neurones which are firing repeatedly. However, it has also been shown that lidocaine has analgesic properties when given systemically (Woolf & Wiesenfeld-Hallin 1985) and that output from some nociceptors can be suppressed without affecting nerve fibre conduction (Tanelian & MacIver 1991). Differential sensory blockade can be achieved by using dilute solutions of the local anaesthetic in the epidural space and many human patients receive analgesic therapy with continuous infusions of these drugs and can still walk.

Of the current amide local anaesthetics, bupivacaine and ropivacaine appear to provide the widest safety margin with respect to a sensory block with minimal interference with motor activity. In people, ropivacaine at 0.1% induced minimal effects on motor function (Zaric et al 1996) while bupivacaine should be used at concentrations less than 0.125%. These low concentrations of local anaesthetics are usually combined with opioids for most effective analgesia. Even though many of these patients can walk it is also recognised that they do have proprioceptive and sensory deficits (Buggy et al 1994).

Opioids

The site of action of epidurally administered opioids is not certain. Systemic absorption can also account for some effects as well as local diffusion into the cord. Opioids injected into the epidural space will diffuse through the dura and penetrate into both the dorsal horn and central horn of the spinal cord. Spinally, they are thought to work at presynaptic sites preventing the release of substance P and on postsynaptic receptors to hyperpolarise the cells. Thus opioids obtund nociception without having any significant effect on motor function. The potency of different opioids, given by this route, has been studied carefully and it is evident that it is not directly related to systemic potency but rather is a function of lipid solubility. As described above, the permeability of the opioid through the meninges is determined by the lipid solubility characteristics but the activity of these drugs when injected into the intrathecal space is also a function of lipid solubility. This relationship is more straightforward with a decreasing potency with increasing lipophilicity (Dickenson et al 1990). The potency in the latter study was measured as the ED_{50} for inhibition of C fibre evoked responses in anaesthetised rats and in this model morphine was more potent than fentanyl (ED_{50} of 15.8 and 85 nmol, respectively). In fact, fentanyl was more effective when given intravenously.

Morphine

This drug has been the most useful opioid to give epidurally because it has a high potency with a long duration of action. In dogs, epidural morphine at 0.1 mg/kg has an onset time of about 20–60 minutes (Bonath & Saleh 1985) and a duration of action of 16–24 hours (Dodman et al 1992, Popilskis et al 1993). It has been used with good effect in cats and dogs (Tung & Yaksh 1982, Popilskis et al 1993). Epidural morphine decreased the MAC of halothane in dogs by at least 40% (Valverde et al 1989) and the MAC of isoflurane in cats by about 30% (Golder et al 1998). Using this technique provided less cardiovascular depression in an experimental setting than using an equivalent dose of inhalant (Valverde et al 1991). In people the common side-effects reported with epidural morphine are pruritus, respiratory depression, urinary retention and nausea. In dogs pruritus does occur but is relatively uncommon, while respiratory depression may develop but seems to have minimal clinical importance. Both of these side-effects are reversible with an opioid antagonist administered systemically – suggesting systemic absorption – but as long as the dose of the antagonist is titrated carefully one can reverse these side-effects without reducing local analgesia. Urinary retention is certainly likely (Drenger & Magora 1989) but has been a minor issue in a clinical environment. A recent case report involving urinary retention in a dog following epidural morphine and bupivacaine shows that it is important to monitor urinary function postoperatively (Herperger 1998). Nausea appears to be uncommon in dogs and cats since vomiting rarely occurs after epidural morphine in these species. Only about 0.3% of the epidural morphine is thought to cross the meninges in dogs (Durant & Yaksh 1986).

In horses morphine has been used at doses of 0.1–0.2 mg/kg diluted in volumes of 20–30 ml of saline for the management of severe hindlimb pain (Valverde et al 1990). Clinically, analgesia appears to occur within 20–30 minutes. In an experimental study the onset times were much longer: 6–8 hours with doses of 0.05–0.10 mg/kg diluted in 10 ml saline (Robinson et al 1994). The differences in onset time may be due to the nociceptive testing methods used in this study – morphine analgesia is not expected to blunt sharp pain as much as the dull, aching, throbbing pain associated with injury – and this study only used needle and electrical nociceptive stimuli. The duration of analgesia in the above study was 9–13 hours after analgesia onset (17–19 hours after injection); and it seems that, clinically, the duration is about 8–16 hours (Valverde et al 1990, Robinson et al 1994). Morphine has also been used in combination with detomidine (0.2 mg/kg morphine + 30 μg/kg detomidine) and provided excellent relief in an induced model of synovitis pain of the tarsocrural joint (Sysel et al 1996) and following bilateral stifle arthroscopy (Goodrich et al 1999). Epidural morphine reduced the MAC of halothane in horses by 14% (Doherty et al 1997).

Meperidine (pethidine)

This drug has both local anaesthetic properties and opioid activity (Jaffe & Rowe 1996). In a study in cats it was shown that meperidine had a rapid onset of action with a duration of 1–4 hours depending on dose (Tung & Yaksh 1982). Its analgesic actions were reversible with naloxone. In people it also has a rapid onset with a duration of action of about 6 hours (Torda & Pybus 1982). Its epidural potency was shown to be 1/35th that of morphine (Sjöström et al 1988).

Methadone

In cats 0.7–1.0 mg/kg gives a rapid onset of action with a duration of about 4 hours (Tung & Yaksh 1982). In people it has a duration of about 9 hours (Torda & Pybus 1982). Epidural methadone was shown to increase bladder tone and decrease bladder compliance in dogs but there appears to be a lower incidence of urinary complications in women when compared with the use of epidural morphine (Evron et al 1985, Drenger et al 1986).

Oxymorphone

This drug has not been used widely in humans but has been used in some canine studies. At 0.1 mg/kg epidurally it was shown to be more effective and lasted significantly longer (10 hours vs 2 hours) than 0.2 mg/kg given i.m. (Popilskis et al 1991). In another study 0.05 mg/kg epidurally gave about 7 hours of analgesia with few side-effects (Vesal et al 1996). It is not clear what the dose of oxymorphone should be since it has a similar lipid solubility to morphine but is 10 times more potent when given systemically.

Fentanyl

There is considerable debate as to whether there is any point in using fentanyl epidurally. It is so highly lipid soluble that its permeability across the meninges is reduced and once it reaches the CSF its potency is much less than would be predicted, such that intravenous fentanyl gives a similar effect (Loper et al 1990). The main use for fentanyl appears to be as an adjunct to other epidural drugs (Fischer et al 1988). When used with morphine there is a faster onset of analgesia, which may be useful if an epidural is being given for acute pain or shortly before the onset of pain (e.g. end of surgery). When used with bupivacaine there seems to be an enhancement of the action of the local anaesthetic.

Sufentanil

Many of the comments about fentanyl apply to sufentanil but it does not appear to have an effect that is greater when given epidurally than when it is given systemically (Rosseel et al 1988). In dogs, lumbar CSF concentrations of sufentanil peaked 6.5 minutes after epidural injection (Stevens et al 1993) so it is expected to have a rapid onset of action. There is some suggestion that sufentanil may have an action at spinal receptors which exceeds that seen with morphine. Patients with a tolerance to epidural morphine were provided with adequate analgesia after sufentanil (de Leon-Casasola & Lema 1994).

Butorphanol

A number of studies have been carried out with this drug and again there is some debate as to whether there is any advantage to administering the drug epidurally rather than intravenously (Camann et al 1992). In a study of intrathecal butorphanol in sheep, there was noticeable neurotoxicity but the adverse effects noted in this study have not been seen in other species (Rawal et al 1991). In combination with lidocaine it prolonged the duration of epidural analgesia in horses (Csik-Salmon et al 1996). The horses were not ataxic but had a peculiar high-stepping gait following this treatment. In dogs at 0.25 mg/kg it has been shown to reduce the MAC of isoflurane by 31% and to have an analgesic action of about 3 hours (Troncy et al 1996). Since this MAC reduction is greater than that reported for systemically administered butorphanol, it would suggest that epidural administration is more effective (Quandt et al 1994). In horses (0.05 mg/kg) it did not change the MAC of halothane (Doherty et al 1997).

Buprenorphine

It has a slow onset of action, reaching its peak effect at about 60 minutes. The analgesic effects appear to be similar to those of epidural morphine with a potency ratio of 8:1 (Chrubasik et al 1987) suggesting that a dose of 12.5 μg/kg would be equivalent to 0.1 mg/kg of morphine. In humans at 4 μg/kg the reduction of the MAC of halothane was equivalent to that observed for a similar i.v. dose (Inagaki & Kuzukawa 1997) but the same authors showed that the analgesia in surgical patients was more intense in the segments affected by the epidural injection than an equivalent i.v. dose (Inagaki et al 1996). The duration of analgesia with epidural buprenorphine is similar to that of morphine (Miwa et al 1996). The occurrence of urinary retention is less likely with buprenorphine since it has minimal effect on urodynamics in dogs (Drenger & Magora 1989).

Alpha-2 agonists

These drugs interact with the adrenergic system in the spinal cord to inhibit the central transmission of nociceptive information. This activity does not appear to be due to the vasoconstriction induced by these drugs. With the alpha-2 agonists alone, it is usual to see sedation as a result of systemic uptake of the drug when epidural doses are given which induce analgesia. The drugs which have been studied most include clonidine, xylazine, detomidine and medetomidine.

Clonidine

This has been used extensively in humans where it has an onset time of about 20 minutes and a dose-dependent duration of action (up to 6 hours). The analgesia produced with clonidine in people is often accompanied by some sedation and systemic hypotension. In sheep, clonidine gives profound analgesia and some sedation with no hypotension (Eisenach et al 1987).

Xylazine

Xylazine has been used extensively in animals and can provide profound analgesia. The chemical structure of xylazine is similar to lidocaine and it has been suggested that some of the action of epidural xylazine is due to this effect. However, it is clear that xylazine can induce analgesia sufficient for surgery without interfering with motor activity in some animals (Caulkett et al 1993). Epidural xylazine (0.75 mg/kg) has been reported to be able to provide surgical analgesia in dogs given 0.5 mg/kg diazepam (Kelawala et al 1996), while at a lower dose (0.25 mg/kg) it provided postoperative analgesia which was not reversible with atipamezole (Rector et al 1998). At an even lower dose (0.02 mg/kg) in combination with epidural morphine (0.1 mg/kg) there was no effect seen on a variety of cardiopulmonary parameters measured during isoflurane anaesthesia (Keegan et al 1995), but no attempt was made to measure analgesia in this study. In horses the perineal region of analgesia may be delineated by an increase in sweating from that area. The onset of analgesia occurs within 10–20 minutes and lasts for 2–3 hours in cattle and llamas; in horses the onset was slower (32 minutes) but the duration may be longer (2.5–3.5 hours) and appears to be longer than with detomidine (Skarda & Muir 1996).

The cardiopulmonary side-effects of epidural xylazine (0.25 mg/kg) are far less noticeable than following detomidine – there is a slight decrease in heart rate and blood pressure with no change in cardiac index (Skarda & Muir 1996). Typically, cattle demonstrate signs of sedation and both horses and cattle may become slightly ataxic. Some cattle have become recumbent with epidural xylazine (L. George, personal communication). There is also a reduction in intestinal activity. It has been shown in cattle that the systemic signs can be antagonised by systemic tolazoline without altering the analgesia in the perineal region (Skarda et al 1990).

Detomidine

Mainly used in horses, detomidine can induce profound analgesia with some proprioceptive deficits and ataxia. At 60 μg/kg, detomidine administered at the first coccygeal interspace induced analgesia up to T14 (Skarda & Muir 1994). The onset of analgesia was within 20 minutes and lasted 2–3 hours. This was accompanied by marked sedation, a reduction in heart rate, cardiac index and respiratory rate and an increase in $PaCO_2$ and blood pressure (Skarda & Muir 1994, 1996). Detomidine has been used in combination with morphine in horses (see section on morphine above). In pigs, massive doses of detoidine (500 μg/kg) did not induce analgesia (Ko et al 1992).

Medetomidine and dexmedetomidine

These are the most potent of the currently available alpha-2 agonists, with dexmedetomidine being the active isomer. In dogs, the ED_{50} for epidural medetomidine to a thermal heat stimulus was $10\,\mu g/kg$ (Sabbe et al 1994). At $15\,\mu g/kg$ there was analgesia following surgery which lasted for 4–8 hours (Vesal et al 1996). The dogs in the latter study had decreased heart rates and some had second degree AV blocks, but they were no more sedated than the animals receiving epidural oxymorphone. There was less respiratory depression with the alpha-2 agonist. In cats $10\,\mu g/kg$ gave an increase in the hindlimb pain threshold from 20 to 245 minutes after injection. Most of the cats vomited after the medetomidine and they all appeared to be mildly sedated. There was an initial increase in blood pressure followed by a decrease after 20 minutes. Heart rate and respiratory rate were both decreased.

NMDA antagonists

These drugs have been used epidurally with mixed results when used alone. Their mode of action is thought mainly to be an effect on 'wind-up' or central hyperalgesia; it is likely that they will be most helpful as part of an analgesic therapy rather than as a sole treatment. Some early studies suggested that ketamine might be neurotoxic but this may be due to the preservative (benzethonium chloride). A recent evaluation using preservative-free ketamine did not demonstrate any toxicity even after repeated injections (Borgbjerg et al 1994). Ketamine has been shown to have activity as a local anaesthetic, an NMDA antagonist, an opioid agonist/antagonist and possibly as a muscarinic antagonist (Hirota & Lambert 1996). These complex interactions make it difficult to determine the specific site of action of ketamine-induced analgesia. In some studies epidural ketamine did not show any analgesic effects or it was determined that the side-effects were sufficiently unpleasant for it not to be an acceptable treatment (Kawana et al 1987, Peat et al 1989). In other instances it has been shown to provide adequate analgesia with minor side-effects (Islas et al 1985, Naguib et al 1986).

Another more potent NMDA antagonist (CPP: 3-(2-carboxypiperazan-4-yl) propyl-1-phosphonic acid) has been tested in the hope that it will provide analgesia with less motor dysfunction. This drug given intrathecally showed a dose–related antinociception for a thermal and formalin test but a bell-shaped dose response in the tail flick test in rats. There was minimal motor dysfunction at the lower doses (Kristensen et al 1994). In one human patient this drug abolished the wind-up associated with neurogenic pain (Kristensen et al 1992).

Ketamine has been shown to reduce the MAC of halothane in horses by 14–17% at 0.8–1.2 mg/kg (Doherty et al 1997). Analgesia following epidural ketamine in horses occurred within 5 minutes and lasted for 30–90 minutes, depending on dose (0.5, 1 and 2 mg/kg) and sites tested (Gomez et al 1998).

Other drugs

Non-steroidal antiinflammatory drugs (NSAIDs) (Wang et al 1994, 1995, Gallivan et al 1999), corticosteroids (Molloy & Benzon 1996), anticholinesterases (Nemirovsky & Niv 1996), purinergic agonists (Rane et al 1998), cholecystokinin antagonists (Watkins et al 1985), inhibitors of nitric oxide synthase (Wong et al 1998, Dolan & Nolan 1999), vasopressin (Thurston et al 1988), oxytocin (Yang 1994) and somatostatin (Mollenholt et al 1990) have all been shown to have analgesic properties when administered epidurally or intrathecally. Some of these drugs have undergone minimal testing for neurotoxicity and there are concerns over their use in clinical patients.

Combinations

The above descriptions have focused on the action of each specific drug. Since these drugs have actions which are mostly separate from each other, it is likely that combinations of different classes of drugs will enhance analgesia. This idea has been tested rigorously and a number of studies, using isobolographic techniques, have shown synergism between these compounds. There is a synergism between local anaesthetic and opioids (Wang et al 1993), alpha-2 agonists and opioids (Monasky et al 1990, Branson et al 1993), local anaesthetics and alpha-2 agonists (Grubb et al 1991, 1993, Gaumann et al 1992), NSAIDs and opioids (Malmberg & Yaksh 1993) and ketamine and μ agonist opioids (Wong et al 1996). These combinations and further additions are being used clinically at doses which minimise the side-effects of each individual drug (see Table 5.1).

Preservatives

There are very few drugs which are marketed for epidural or spinal use. Many of the drugs discussed above are available in preparations designed for systemic use and contain preservatives. The neurotoxicity of these preservatives is largely untested. There have been concerns expressed over sodium bisulphite, benzethonium chloride, chlorbutanol and disodium EDTA (Olek & Edwards 1980, Ford & Raj 1987, Wang et al 1992, Yaksh 1996). Methyl paraben does not appear to be neurotoxic although in people it is associated with allergic responses (Adams et al 1977).

Air

In testing for needle placement in the epidural space many people use a 'loss of resistance' technique, injecting a small quantity of air into the epidural space.

While small quantities of air are unlikely to be detrimental, larger volumes may be associated with incomplete or patchy absorption of epidural drugs, neurological deficits and even air embolism (Dales et al 1987, Deam & Scott 1993, Sethna & Berde 1993). It should also be remembered that the administration of N_2O after injection of air epidurally will lead to an increase in the size of the bubbles, with possible increases in pressure on the spinal cord (Stevens et al 1989).

Local anaesthetic agents and dose rates

The most commonly used local anaesthetics are lidocaine and bupivacaine. Lidocaine has a rapid onset (1–2 minutes) and short duration (1.5–2.0 hours) of action. Bupivacaine has a slower onset of action (5–10 minutes), but a much longer duration (4–12 hours, depending upon the site). Both drugs can be associated with toxic effects, especially after inadvertent intravenous injection. Intravenous administration of lidocaine or bupivacaine can cause hypotension, dysrhythmias, e.g. atrioventricular block, and central nervous system depression followed by seizures. With both drugs, sedation is seen first, then agitation, restlessness, vomiting and then seizure activity and finally complete CNS depression. Both are toxic to tissues, but this is of little clinical relevance unless other factors are present to delay healing. Bupivacaine has more marked cardiotoxic effects than lidocaine. Toxic doses are 10–20 mg/kg for lidocaine and 4 mg/kg for bupivacaine, given intravenously, and so maximum safe doses for most species are:

> 4 mg/kg lidocaine (0.4 ml/kg of 1% solution)
> 1–2 mg/kg bupivacaine (0.4–0.8 ml/kg of 0.25% solution)

These doses should be diluted to provide an appropriate volume, e.g. in a 3 kg cat receiving an intercostal block with bupivacaine, 1 ml of 0.25% solution can be diluted to 4 ml and approximately 0.8 ml injected at each site. Aspiration should always be performed prior to injection and care should be taken when dosing small dogs, cats and small mammals with local anaesthetic as their small size increases the risk of overdose. It is always advisable to weigh the animal and calculate the maximum safe dose accurately as quite a small error in estimation of the bodyweight in these small animals often results in serious consequences.

Local anaesthetics are available in a variety of concentrations with or without adrenaline (1:100000 or 1:200000 dilutions of adrenaline). Adrenaline causes vasoconstriction and prolongs the action of the local anaesthetic. Local anaesthetic without adrenaline should be used in high–risk patients to avoid any possibility of cardiac stimulation and when performing 'ring blocks' of appendages.

Local anaesthetics have been administered in small doses intravenously to provide postoperative analgesia (Cassuto et al 1985) and for cancer pain in man. So far there have been few reports of the use of this technique in animals, although lidocaine infusions have been shown to decrease MAC (Doherty & Frazier

Opioid analgesic	Dog	Cat
Buprenorphine	0.005–0.020 mg/kg i.m., s.c. or i.v.; 6–12 hourly	0.005–0.020 mg/kg i.m., s.c. or i.v.; 6–12 hourly
Butorphanol	0.2–0.6 mg/kg i.m., s.c. or i.v.; 2–4 hourly	0.2–0.8 mg/kg i.m. or s.c.; 2–4 hourly
Fentanyl	0.001–0.005 mg/kg i.v. repeated every 20–30 minutes, or by continuous infusion (0.003–0.010 mg/kg/h)	?
Methadone	0.10–0.25 mg/kg i.m., s.c. or i.v.; 4–6 hourly	?
Morphine	0.1–1.0 mg/kg i.m., s.c. or i.v.; 4–6 hourly	0.1–0.2 mg/kg i.m., s.c. or i.v.; 6–8 hourly
Nalbuphine	0.3–0.5 mg/kg i.m., s.c.; 3–4 hourly	0.3–0.5 mg/kg i.m., s.c. or i.v.; 3 hourly
Oxymorphone	0.05–0.20 mg/kg i.m., s.c. or i.v.; 2–4 hourly	0.05–0.40 mg/kg i.m., s.c. or i.v.; 2–4 hourly
Papaveretum	0.2–0.8 mg/kg i.m. or i.v.; ? 4 hourly	0.1–0.3 mg/kg i.m.; ?4 hourly
Pentazocine	1–4 mg/kg i.m. or i.v.; 2–4 hourly	1–4 mg/kg i.m. or i.v.; 2–3 hourly
Pethidine (meperidine)	3.5–10.0 mg/kg i.m. or 10–15 mg/kg s.c.; 2.5–3.5 hourly	3.5–10.0 mg/kg i.m. or 10–15 mg/kg s.c.; 2–3 hourly
Naloxone (antagonist)	0.04–1.00 mg/kg i.m., s.c. or i.v.	0.04–1.00 mg/kg i.m., s.c. or i.v.

Table 5.2 Opioid analgesics for use in the dog and cat. Dose rates are based on published data and the clinical experience of the authors. Dose should be adjusted to produce the desired effect, and administration repeated as needed to control pain. Particular care should be taken when administering these drugs by the intravenous route, as rapid administration can lead to inadvertent overdose.

1998) and the technique has been used clinically (see below). It has also been suggested that intravenous lidocaine can be of value for pain relief in conditions such as laminitis and colic in horses (P. Taylor, personal communication).

Clinical assessment of the effects of intravenous lidocaine in the horse suggest that it provides mild visceral analgesia. It should be administered as an initial loading dose of 1.3 mg/kg i.v. followed by a continuous infusion of 0.05 mg/kg i.v. The continuous infusion is conveniently administered by adding 550 ml of 2% lidocaine to 5 L of balanced electrolyte solution, providing a 2 mg/ml solution. This solution is stable for 21 days. Initial studies indicate that the toxic serum level is between 1.5 and 4.5 μg/ml. The target plasma concentration for analgesia is around 1.0 μg/ml. Clinical signs of toxicity are skeletal muscle fasciculations followed by ataxia and then collapse. Discontinuation of administration will generally result in resolution of these signs within 5–10 minutes. The half-life of lidocaine in the horse is 39.8 minutes. Four days of lidocaine treatment resulted in no alterations in serum chemistry, ECG parameters, or haematology outside of normal values during the treatment period (Meyer, personal communication).

Perioperative use of analgesics – practical considerations

Dosages are given in Tables 5.2–5.9. After considering all of the points discussed above, the following key practical points should be noted:

Severe pain

- If severe intractable pain occurs immediately postoperatively, remember that re-establishing general anaesthesia will prevent the animal experiencing pain while a more effective analgesic protocol is implemented.

Opioids (Tables 5.2–5.5)

- Partial agonists (buprenorphine) and mixed agonist-antagonists (butorphanol) have a maximal effect. This will be produced in most animals by the upper end of the doses listed in Tables 5.2–5.5. If analgesia is inadequate, additional doses are less likely to be effective than changing to the use of a pure μ agonist (e.g. morphine, oxymorphone or methadone) or alternative therapies (e.g. local block, epidural or intrathecal opioids).
- In clinical use there is no upper limit to the analgesia available with pure μ agonists (e.g. morphine, oxymorphone, pethidine, methadone). The major limiting factor to their use is respiratory depression, although this is rarely seen until doses are administered that are much higher than those normally used clinically. In horses, there is a significant risk of excitement if morphine is administered, unless sedatives are administered concurrently; butorphanol is recommended in this species.
- The main role of opioids is to provide relief from severe pain, and to supplement the analgesia provided by NSAIDs. Repeated increments can be given as needed, when pain appears to be returning. For extended postoperative pain relief, where NSAIDs alone prove inadequate, morphine can be given as sustained release tablets in dogs, or fentanyl patches may be used (see chapter 7).
- Consider administering opioids by continuous infusion (see above) to provide more effective, sustained pain relief.

NSAIDs (Tables 5.6–5.9)

- In general, manufacturers currently recommend these should be given as a single dose at the end of anaesthesia, or in the recovery phase, with the exception of carprofen. As additional information on safety is obtained, it

Opioid analgesic	Ferret	Guinea pig	Mouse	Rat	Rabbit
Buprenorphine	0.01–0.03 mg/kg i.m., s.c. or i.v.; 6–12 hourly	0.05 mg/kg s.c.; 8–12 hourly	0.05–0.10 mg/kg s.c.; 8–12 hourly	0.01–0.05 mg/kg s.c. or i.v.; 8–12 hourly / 0.10–0.25 mg/kg by mouth; 8–12 hourly	0.01–0.05 mg/kg i.m., s.c. or i.v.; 6–12 hourly
Butorphanol	0.4 mg/kg i.m.; 4 hourly	?	1.0–2.0 mg/kg i.m. or s.c.; 4 hourly	1.0–2.0 mg/kg i.m. or s.c.; 2–4 hourly	0.1–0.5 mg/kg i.m., s.c. or i.v.; 4 hourly
Morphine	0.5–2.0 mg/kg i.m., s.c.; 4–6 hourly	2–5 mg/kg i.m., s.c.; 4 hourly	2–5 mg/kg i.m., s.c.; 4 hourly	2–5 mg/kg i.m., s.c.; 4 hourly	2–5 mg/kg i.m., s.c.; 4 hourly
Nalbuphine	?	1–2 mg/kg i.m.; 4 hourly	2–4 mg/kg i.m.; 4 hourly	1–2 mg/kg i.m.; 4 hourly	1–2 mg/kg i.m.; i.v.; 4 hourly
Pentazocine	?	?	5–10 mg/kg s.c. or i.m.; 3–4 hourly	5–10 mg/kg s.c. or i.m.; 3–4 hourly	5–10 mg/kg s.c., i.m. or i.v.; 4 hourly
Pethidine (meperidine)	5–10 mg/kg i.m.; 2–4 hourly	10 mg/kg i.m.; 2–4 hourly	10–20 mg/kg s.c. or i.m.; 2–3 hourly	10–20 mg/kg s.c. or i.m.; 2–3 hourly	5–10 mg/kg s.c. or i.m.; 2–3 hourly
Naloxone (antagonist)	0.04–1.00 mg/kg i.m., s.c. or i.v.	?	?	0.01–0.1 mg/kg i.m., s.c. or i.v.	?

Table 5.3 Opioid analgesics for use in rabbits, ferrets and small rodents. Dose rates are based on published data and the clinical experience of the authors. Dose should be adjusted to produce the desired effect, and administration repeated as needed to control pain. Particular care should be taken when administering these drugs by the intravenous route, as rapid administration can lead to inadvertent overdose. No good data are available concerning suitable dose rates for gerbils or hamsters, but clinical experience suggests that dose rates indicated for rats are appropriate.

Opioid analgesic	Cow	Goat	Horse	Pig	Sheep
Buprenorphine	?	0.005 mg/kg i.m.; 12 hourly	0.004–0.006 mg/kg .i.v.	0.005–0.050 mg/kg i.v. or i.m.; 6–12 hourly	0.005–0.010 mg/kg i.v. or i.m.; 4 hourly
Butorphanol	?	0.5 mg/kg i.m. or s.c.; 2–3 hourly	0.05–0.10 mg/kg i.v. or i.m.; 8 hourly	0.1–0.3 mg/kg i.m.; 4 hourly	0.5 mg/kg i.m. or s.c.; 2–3 hourly
Methadone	?	?	0.1 mg/kg i.m.; 4 hourly	?	?
Morphine	?	0.2–0.5 mg/kg i.m.	0.1 mg/kg i.m.; 4 hourly	0.2–1.0 mg/kg i.m.; ?4 hourly	0.2–0.5 mg/kg i.m.; ? 2 hourly
Oxymorphone	?	?	?	0.02 mg/kg i.m.	?
Pentazocine	?	?	?	2 mg/kg i.m. or i.v.; 4 hourly	?
Pethidine (meperidine)	?	?	1–2 mg/kg i.m.; 1–2 hourly	2 mg/kg i.m. or i.v.; 2–4 hourly	2 mg/kg i.m. or i.v.; 2 hourly

Table 5.4 Opioid analgesics for use in horses and farm animals. Dose rates are based on published data (Flecknell 1996, Wolfensohn & Lloyd 1998, Thurmon et al 1996) and the clinical experience of the authors. Dose should be adjusted to produce the desired effect, and administration repeated as needed to control pain. Particular care should be taken when administering these drugs by the intravenous route, as rapid administration can lead to inadvertent overdose.

Opioid analgesic	Non-human primates	Birds	Reptiles
Buprenorphine	0.005–0.010 mg/kg i.m., s.c. or i.v.; 6–12 hourly	0.01–0.05 mg/kg i.m.	0.01 mg/kg i.m.
Butorphanol	0.01 mg/kg i.v.; ?3–4 hourly	1–4 mg/kg i.m.; 2–4 hourly (psittacines)	25 mg/kg i.m. (tortoises)
Morphine	0.1–2.0 mg/kg i.m., s.c. or i.v.; 4–6 hourly	?	?
Pentazocine	2–4 mg/kg i.m. or i.v.; 2–4 hourly	?	?
Pethidine (meperidene)	2–4 mg/kg i.m.; 2–3 hourly	? ?	20 mg/kg i.m.; 12–24 hourly (tortoises)

Table 5.5 Opioid analgesics for use in other species. Dose rates are based on published data (Clyde & Paul-Murphy 1998, Thurmon et al 1996, Malley 1999) and the clinical experience of the authors. Dose should be adjusted to produce the desired effect, and administration repeated as needed to control pain. Particular care should be taken when administering these drugs by the intravenous route, as rapid administration can lead to inadvertent overdose.

may be possible to use the more effective technique of preoperative administration with a wider range of agents.

- These agents are best considered as 'single-shot' analgesics, with no real facility to titrate the dose against the severity of the pain. Onset of action is relatively slow, so a 'top-up' dose in cases of inadequate analgesia will have a delayed effect. In these circumstances an opioid is often preferable.
- The slow onset of action can lead to a gap in pain relief, especially when the NSAID is given postoperatively. To avoid this 'pain breakthrough', use an additional analgesic (e.g. an opioid) preoperatively or during recovery. Pethidine (meperidine) is useful for this purpose in many species, and butorphanol in farm animals and horses.
- For some surgical procedures, NSAIDs may be sufficiently effective so that no supplementary analgesia will be needed once the NSAID has reached its peak effect. Oral NSAIDs are ideal for extending the period of postoperative pain control for several days.

Analgesic treatment of other acute pain

The general principles discussed above in relation to perioperative and trauma pain also apply to other conditions in which acute pain occurs. Controlling pain associated with neoplasia is discussed in chapter 7. The following practical points should be considered:

- It is important to treat the underlying disease at the same time as controlling pain.

NSAIDs and mild analgesics	Cat	Dog
Acetylsalicylic acid	10–25 mg/kg by mouth every 48 hours	10–25 mg/kg by mouth every 8–12 hours
Carprofen	2–4 mg/kg s.c. or i.v., single dose; 2 mg/kg orally for 4 days, then every other day (well-tolerated long term)	4 mg/kg s.c. or i.v., single dose; 4 mg/kg orally (well-tolerated long term)
Dipyrone (in 'Buscopan Compositum') (500 mg/ml)		1.0–2.5 ml/kg i.v. or i.m.
Flunixin	1 mg/kg s.c. or slow i.v., single dose; 1 mg/kg orally, single dose	1 mg/kg s.c. or slow i.v., single dose; 1 mg/kg orally, daily for up to 3 days
Ketoprofen	2 mg/kg s.c., daily for up to 3 days; 1 mg/kg orally, daily for up to 5 days	2 mg/kg s.c., daily for up to 3 days; 1 mg/kg orally, daily for up to 5 days
Meloxicam	0.2 mg/kg s.c., single dose; 0.3 mg/kg orally on day 1, then 0.1 mg/kg orally daily for 3 days, then 0.1 mg/cat daily	0.2 mg/kg s.c., single dose; 0.2 mg/kg orally on day 1, then 0.1 mg/kg orally daily (well-tolerated long term)
Paracetamol (acetominophen)	Contraindicated	15 mg/kg by mouth 6–8 hourly
Phenylbutazone	1 × 25 mg tablet twice daily for up to 5 days; to 1 × 25 mg daily (high maintenance dose) or 1 × 25 mg every other day (low maintenance dose) – all doses for 3.5 kg cat	2–20 mg/kg daily for up to 7 days, then reduce to lowest effective dose
Tolfenamic acid	4 mg/kg s.c., daily for up to 2 days; 4 mg/kg orally, daily for up to 3 days	4 mg/kg s.c. every 24 hours for up to 2 days; 4 mg/kg orally, daily for up to 3 days

Table 5.6 NSAID and other analgesics for use in the dog and cat. Dose rates are based on published data and the clinical experience of the authors. Refer to the text for contraindications and precautions to be observed, particularly for long-term administration.

- When dealing with inflammatory disease processes, NSAIDs will be useful, but do not overlook their potential interactions with corticosteroids. This is unlikely to be a problem in short-term therapy, but may be of significant concern if therapy is prolonged (see chapter 3).
- Use of local anaesthesia, especially where regional blocks are suitable, is often overlooked as a means of controlling pain associated with many medical diseases.

NSAIDs and mild analgesics	Ferret	Guinea pig	Mouse	Rat	Rabbit
Acetylsalicylic acid	20 mg/kg by mouth, ?once	80–90 mg/kg by mouth, ?once	120 mg/kg by mouth, ?once	100 mg/kg by mouth, ?once	100 mg/kg by mouth, ?once
Carprofen	?	?	5 mg/kg s.c. or by mouth daily	5 mg/kg s.c. or by mouth daily	4 mg/kg s.c., daily or 1.5 mg/kg by mouth, b.i.d.
Diclofenac	?	2.0 mg/kg by mouth daily	8.0 mg/kg by mouth daily	10 mg/kg by mouth daily	?
Flunixin	0.5–2.0 mg/kg s.c.; 12–24 hourly	?	2.5 mg/kg s.c.; ? 12–24 hourly	2.5 mg/kg s.c.; ? 12–24 hourly	1.0 mg/kg s.c.; ? 12–24 hourly
Ibuprofen	?	?	30 mg/kg by mouth daily	15 mg/kg by mouth daily	?
Ketoprofen	?	?	?	5 mg/kg s.c. or by mouth daily	3 mg/kg s.c. daily
Meloxicam	?	?	?	1.0 mg/kg s.c. or by mouth daily	0.2 mg/kg s.c. daily ?up to 3 days
Paracetamol (acetaminophen)	?	?	200 mg/kg by mouth, ?daily	200 mg/kg by mouth, ?daily	?
Piroxicam	?	6 mg/kg by mouth, ?daily	3 mg/kg by mouth, ?daily	3 mg/kg by mouth, ?daily	0.2 mg/kg by mouth, t.i.d.

Table 5.7 NSAID and other analgesics for use in rabbits, ferrets and small rodents. Dose rates are based on published data and the clinical experience of the authors. Refer to the text for contraindications and precautions to be observed, particularly for long-term administration. No good data are available concerning suitable dose rates for gerbils or hamsters, but clinical experience suggests that dose rates indicated for rats are appropriate.

NSAIDs and mild analgesics	Cow	Goat	Horse	Pig	Sheep
Acetylsalicylic acid	?	?	25 mg/kg by mouth 12 hourly, twice; then 10 mg/kg daily	10 mg/kg by mouth; 4 hourly	50–100 mg/kg by mouth; 6–12 hourly
Carprofen	1.4 mg/kg s.c. or i.v., single dose	?	0.7 mg/kg i.v. daily (2 doses max.); 0.7 mg/kg by mouth daily for 4–9 days	2–4 mg/kg s.c. or i.v. daily	1.5–2.0 mg/kg s.c. or i.v. daily
Flunixin	2.2 mg/kg i.v. daily for up to 5 days	1 mg/kg once	1.1 mg/kg by mouth or i.v. daily for up to 5 days	1–2 mg/kg s.c. or i.v. daily	2 mg/kg s.c. or i.v. daily
Ketoprofen	3 mg/kg i.m. or i.v. daily for up to 3 days	?	2.2 mg/kg i.v. daily for up to 5 days	3 mg/kg i.m. once	?
Meloxicam	0.5 mg/kg s.c. or i.v. one dose (active for 3 days)	?	?	?	?
Phenylbutazone	?	?	4.4 mg/kg by mouth b.i.d. for 1 day, then 2.2 mg/kg b.i.d. for 2–4 days, then 2.2 mg/kg on alternate days	?	?10 mg/kg by mouth
Tolfenamic acid	2 mg/kg i.m. once daily	?	?	?	?

Table 5.8 NSAID and other analgesics for use in horses and farm animals. Dose rates are based on published data (Bishop 1998, Thurmon et al 1996) and the clinical experience of the authors. Refer to the text for contraindications and precautions to be observed, particularly for long-term administration.

NSAIDS and mild analgesics	Non-human primates	Birds	Reptiles
Acetylsalicylic acid	20 mg/kg by mouth; 6–8 hourly	5 mg/kg by mouth 6–8 hourly; or 325 mg/250 ml drinking water	?
Carprofen	3–4 mg/kg s.c. daily for up to 3 days	1–4 mg/kg i.m.	2–4 mg/kg s.c., i.v., i.m. or by mouth once, then 1–2 mg/kg 24–72 hourly
Flunixin	0.5–4.0 mg/kg s.c. or i.v. daily	1–10 mg/kg i.m. daily	0.1–0.5 mg/kg i.m. or i.v. 12–24 hourly for 1–2 days
Ketoprofen	2 mg/kg s.c. daily	2–4 mg/kg i.m.	2 mg/kg s.c. or i.m. every 1–2 days
Meloxicam	?	?	0.1–0.2 mg/kg by mouth daily

Table 5.9 NSAID and other analgesics for use in other species. Dose rates are based on published data (Wolfensohn & Lloyd 1998, Malley 1999) and the clinical experience of the authors. Refer to the text for contraindications and precautions to be observed, particularly for long-term administration.

- Topical local anaesthetic may be useful.
- As with other acute pain, use NSAIDs and opioids concurrently if pain is severe, or when immediate pain relief is required (provided by the opioid), followed by more sustained analgesia (provided by the NSAID).
- As with pain associated with trauma, immobilising the affected area will often reduce the degree of pain.
- Sedation may enhance analgesia by preventing anxiety and fear.

Specific clinical examples

Otitis externa

Pain associated with this condition can be severe, and although medical or surgical treatment usually resolves the primary problem, the pain can persist for several days. Topical preparations containing local anaesthetic are of value, but concurrent administration of systemic NSAIDs and, in cases of severe pain, opioids are also beneficial. Use of sedatives to reduce panic may also be required and can reduce the discomfort associated with the condition and break the cycle of self-trauma.

Ocular disease, e.g. corneal ulcer, acute conjunctivitis, distichiasis and keratitis

As with most conditions, medical or other therapy will resolve the condition, but these conditions can be intensely painful, and the pain may cause a cycle of self-trauma that exacerbates the problem. Topical local anaesthetics are of particular value in preventing the secondary injury arising from self-trauma. Both NSAIDs and opioids can also be used, depending upon the severity of the pain. Retrobulbar nerve block can be used to control severe intractable pain, but the risk of damage to vital structures is high and the block is technically quite difficult to perform safely. Additional measures, such as protection of the eye using a bandage, and bandaging of the foot to reduce self-trauma can also be useful.

Nasal conditions (e.g. foreign body, neoplasia, aspergillus infection)

Topical nasal sprays of local anaesthetic to reduce sneezing and self-trauma caused by rubbing and scratching (e.g. after foreign body removal) can be useful. Systemic NSAIDs and opioids may be required, together with sedatives to reduce fear and panic. Alpha-2 agonists such as medetomidine are also effective and reduce the incidence of sneezing after rhinoscopy or foreign body removal (Pascoe 1999, personal communication).

Colic and other gastrointestinal conditions

Horse: It is clearly of primary importance to establish an accurate diagnosis, and the nature, location and intensity of pain may be an important diagnostic tool. However, short-acting analgesics (e.g. butorphanol, pethidine, Buscopan, or a short-acting alpha-2 adrenoreceptor agonist) can be administered if the animal is being transported to a referral centre, although clearly it is important to consult with the receiving clinician.

Once a definitive diagnosis has been established, or a decision made to carry out surgery, then an NSAID should be administered to provide analgesia. In addition, as discussed earlier, these drugs inhibit cyclooxygenase, whose products mediate many of the clinical effects of endotoxaemia. Flunixin appears particularly effective in this respect. Further details of the management of colic in horses is given in chapter 7.

Dog: As with the horse, establishing a diagnosis is important, but drugs with a short latency may be needed during this period simply to carry out a full examination. Opioids are usually required, but avoid the use of opioids that cause biliary or pancreatic duct spasm, so use of butorphanol, buprenorphine or pethidine is particularly recommended. Management of pancreatitis is discussed in chapter 7.

Musculoskeletal (e.g. myopathies, arthritis)

Generally, NSAIDs are most effective for controlling the pain associated with muscle ischaemia in animals with myopathy, but occasionally opioids are required, as well as sedatives to control fear and panic. When managing arthritis in dogs, it is advisable not to use NSAIDs and corticosteroids concurrently.

Skin (dermatitis, burns)

NSAIDs are particularly valuable if there is severe skin damage resulting in prostaglandin release. Topical local anaesthetics can also be used, and opioids if pain is severe. As with other painful conditions, sedatives may be helpful if the animal is panicking (see chapter 7).

Obstetrics

Some pain is inevitably associated with normal parturition, but it is not considered practical or desirable to administer analgesics routinely to parturient animals. However, when pain becomes excessive because of dystocia, particularly when a decision has been made to carry out a Caesarean section, further pain should be prevented by administration of opioids or NSAIDs. Following parturition, if an animal develops mastitis, current therapeutic regimens rarely include the use of analgesics. This is an obviously painful condition, and use of analgesics will encourage the dam to continue to nurse her offspring while other therapy resolves the primary condition. If high doses of opioids have been given prior to parturition or Caesarean section, then this can potentially depress respiratory function in the offspring. If this appears to be a problem, then respiration can be stimulated using doxapram, and the opioid reversed by administration of naloxone. Although opioids can be transferred into milk, these have no clinically significant effect in the newborn animals because of the low concentrations in the milk and low efficacy of these drugs when administered orally.

The conditions discussed above are by no means an exhaustive list of the situations in which pain could occur. When not contraindicated because of other factors, pain should be treated, in addition to implementing therapy to resolve the underlying cause.

Adjuncts to pain relief

In concentrating on analgesic regimens, and developing ever more appropriate and effective protocols, it is easy to overlook the importance of other factors in managing postoperative and other acute pain. When carrying out surgical procedures, gentle handling of tissues, and careful techniques that minimise tissue trauma will result in less nociceptive stimulation, and so reduce central sensitisation. In addition, good surgical technique which minimises tissue trauma and the prevention of tension on suture lines can considerably reduce the degree of post-surgical pain. The use of bandages to pad and protect traumatised tissue must not be overlooked and forms an essential adjunct to the use of analgesic drugs. Similarly, splinting to reduce movement at the site of injury can also be of value.

Many animals will respond positively to human contact, and nursing care, and stroking, grooming, and other forms of attention can be a useful adjunct to analgesic therapy. The response varies both between individual animals, and between species, and an appropriate level of care and attention must be selected. For example, most dogs and many cats respond positively to such attention, while small mammals and rabbits often find it stressful.

Provision of the most appropriate environmental conditions for recovery from surgery will also improve the general comfort of the patient, reduce fear and anxiety, and so is likely to reduce the degree of pain experienced. Ensuring animals are maintained at an appropriate environmental temperature, have comfortable bedding, and do not become soiled with urine and faeces are all important adjuncts in managing postoperative pain. Dogs and cats may also suffer discomfort if they develop a full bladder, and are reluctant to urinate because of inability to adopt a normal stance, because of pain, or due to the unfamiliar surroundings. If necessary, the bladder should be catheterised to prevent or relieve this discomfort. Ensuring the animal recovers from anaesthesia with an empty bladder will encourage it to rest quietly, and not attempt to stand (to urinate) too rapidly. This is particularly important in the horse.

Fear and anxiety increase the degree of pain perceived in man and increases the requirement for analgesic therapy (Chapman 1985). It is likely that similar effects occur in animals, so measures to minimise fear and anxiety should be considered an essential part of nursing care. This aspect of pain management is often neglected. It is easy to overlook the effects on a small rodent or rabbit of housing it in close proximity to a predator such as a cat or dog. Similarly, a cat being nursed in the same room as a barking, aggressive dog is likely to be fearful and apprehensive. In addition to preventing direct interaction between patients, animals may also be affected by the odours remaining in the cage or recovery pen, or by odours on the clinicians hands or clothing. This can be prevented by effective cleaning of pens, and by carrying out nursing procedures on 'prey' species before dealing with 'predators'.

Analgesic protocols for different species

Dogs

NSAIDs

Dogs are particularly sensitive to the adverse renal effects of NSAIDs during periods of hypotension. They are also sensitive to the gastrointestinal effects of some NSAIDs (see chapters 3, 6 and 7) and they should be monitored particularly carefully if prolonged administration is contemplated. If signs of haemorrhage develop, e.g. vomiting of blood, melaena, pale mucus membranes, or general signs of depression, then therapy should be discontinued while the cause is determined.

Opioids

Dogs are sensitive to the emetic effects of morphine if used as preanaesthetic medication, but vomiting is rarely seen as a complication when morphine is administered to dogs which are in pain postoperatively. Intravenous administration rarely causes histamine release in dogs, but when this occurs the consequent hypotension can be severe. Morphine is very effective for the control of severe pain in dogs; however, it does not have a veterinary product licence in the UK or USA.

Methadone and oxymorphone both have a medium duration of action in dogs (approximately 2–4 hours) and are effective for controlling severe pain. They have the advantage of rarely causing vomiting, and causing minimal histamine release.

Pethidine (meperidine) is a reliable, but short-acting (60–90 minutes) analgesic in dogs after intramuscular administration, although its duration of action is more prolonged postoperatively due to a decreased rate of hepatic metabolism (Waterman & Kalthum 1989). Subcutaneous administration in this species at recommended doses does not produce effective analgesia (Waterman & Kalthum 1989). Intravenous administration of pethidine can result in severe hypotension due to histamine release.

Buprenorphine is licensed in the UK for use in dogs. The manufacturer's data sheet suggests a duration of action of 12 hours and specifically contraindicates repeat doses before this time has elapsed. There are no published data to support these recommendations, and 4–6 hours is widely recognised as the clinically useful duration of action. In the authors' experience, administration of additional doses at 6–8 hourly intervals for 24–48 hours has not been associated with undesirable effects.

Other agents

Ketamine at normal anaesthetic doses cannot be used alone in dogs without additional drugs to control its extrapyramidal and proconvulsive effects. Either benzodiazepines, which are not invariably effective, or alpha-2 adrenoreceptor agonists, which markedly enhance analgesia but may result in general anaesthesia and have adverse effects on circulatory function, can be used (Cullen 1996). Low doses of ketamine (0.1–1 mg/kg) can be used alone in dogs, and it has been shown to have good, but short-lasting analgesic properties postoperatively. It has potential for preventing hyperalgesia some 10–12 hours post-administration (Slingsby & Waterman-Pearson 1999).

Cats

NSAIDs

Cats have an increased susceptibility to the toxic effects of aspirin and some other NSAIDs. Although problems can be avoided by using appropriate dosing intervals, additional care should be taken when using NSAIDs in this species. At the time of writing, carprofen has a veterinary product licence in the UK for administration by injection of a single, preoperative dose in the cat. The manufacturer provides no indications for repeated doses or oral administration; however, a number of clinicians have routinely administered one additional dose at 24 hours. Oral carprofen has also been used at a dose of 2 mg/kg once daily for 4 days, followed by administration every other day, or even less frequently, for the control of chronic painful conditions. There appears to be considerable individual variation in susceptibility to unwanted side-effects, and on some occasions, individual animals have developed signs of toxicity after only a brief (2–3 day) period of treatment. Information concerning extended use of other NSAIDs (meloxicam and ketoprofen) are similarly limited. Preliminary recommendations are to give meloxicam at 0.3 mg/kg on day 1, followed by 0.1 mg/kg for 3 days, then 0.1 mg/cat daily thereafter.

Opioids

Despite the well-established folklore that opioids cannot be used in cats, all classes of opioids can be administered safely to provide analgesia in this species. Morphine is very effective, with a duration of action of approximately 4 hours. Even in cats which are not experiencing pain, dose rates of 10 times the usual clinical dose are normally required to produce minor behavioural disturbances such as restlessness. Very high doses of around 20 times those used clinically (20 mg/kg) are needed to produce excitement in most cats (see chapter 7). Methadone and oxymorphone can also be used safely in cats, and provide effective analgesia. Butorphanol provides moderate analgesia, but its duration of action appears variable (see chapter 3).

There are no laboratory data on the efficacy and duration of action of buprenorphine in the cat, but clinical experience and results of clinical trials indicate it is a safe and effective drug, with a duration of action of 6–8 hours, at a dose rate of 0.01 mg/kg (Stanway et al 1996, Slingsby & Waterman-Pearson 1998). Repeated doses at 6–8 hourly intervals for 24 hours do not appear to cause undesirable effects. Some cats become markedly sedated with buprenorphine. Buprenorphine and other opioids may cause euphoria, dysphoria, or be hallucinogenic in some individuals. These mood-altering effects can also be seen in other species.

Horses

NSAIDs

NSAIDs have been used successfully in horses for many years and provide effective postoperative analgesia. They are routinely given intravenously before or during anaesthesia, so that they will be effective during surgery as well as during the recovery period. Some preparations (e.g. phenylbutazone) may affect the cardiovascular system, so intravenous administration should be slow. In addition, they may displace anaesthetic drugs from plasma protein binding sites, thus deepening anaesthesia if given rapidly. Although most NSAIDs inhibit prostaglandin synthesis and have been associated with postoperative renal damage in the dog, particularly after hypotensive anaesthesia, this does not appear to be a problem in horses. This is surprising in view of the fact that horses often develop marked hypotension during inhalation anaesthesia, but probably reflects a different control mechanism governing renal blood flow in this species.

NSAIDs are also commonly used during and after colic surgery for their effects on mediators of endotoxaemic symptoms by inhibition of cyclooxygenase (King & Gerring 1989, Taylor & Clarke 1999).

Opioids

Both pure μ and mixed agonist/antagonist opioids are used in horses. They produce little sedation when used alone but in combination with small doses of sedatives they provide chemical restraint with analgesia (see Table 5.4). Opioid-induced respiratory depression and reduced gut motility are rarely a problem in horses when the drugs are used at clinical doses. However, long-term use of opioids may increase intestinal transit time and will occasionally lead to impaction colic after a few days continuous use.

Excitation and stereotypic behaviour, a μ agonist effect, is a significant problem in horses, particularly with morphine. A number of signs may be seen: muscular twitching, particularly around the muzzle, uncontrollable walking, head shaking, cribbing, or simply violent behaviour (Kamerling et al 1985, Mama et al 1992, Taylor & Clarke 1999). Excitement is dose dependent, and is more common following intravenous than intramuscular injection. Excitement is prevented or significantly reduced if low doses of opioids are used in combination with sedatives (see Table 5.10). Opioid-induced excitement in horses is not cortical in origin and may be related to dopamine release in the midbrain or even spinal cord (Tobin 1978, Johnson & Taylor 1997). However, attempts to block locomotor activity with dopamine antagonists have not been successful as the antagonists themselves cause extrapyramidal excitement (Pascoe & Taylor 1997). Acepromazine, widely used as a sedative in conjunction with opioids, itself has dopaminergic antagonist properties and appears to suppress excitement better than more specific dopamine antagonists.

The μ agonist opioids can be reversed by opiate antagonists such as naloxone, naltrexone and nalmefene. This is rarely required when normal therapeutic doses are used but all these have been safely used in horses.

Pethidine (meperidine) (1–2 mg/kg), given intramuscularly, provides good analgesia for 1–2 hours in horses. It is a visceral spasmolytic, so is an excellent analgesic for spasmodic colic. Anaphylactoid reactions occasionally occur if pethidine is given intravenously. The μ agonists such as morphine (0.1 mg/kg) and methadone (0.1 mg/kg) are less commonly used on their own for analgesia, but if used i.m. they provide useful postoperative analgesia for about 4 hours.

Butorphanol has been reported occasionally to cause excitement in horses, but this is rarely a clinical problem in horses in pain. Butorphanol (0.05–0.10

Drug combination	Dog	Cat	Horse
Acepromazine Buprenorphine	0.05 mg/kg i.m. 0.01 mg/kg i.m.	0.05 mg/kg i.m. 0.01 mg/kg i.m.	–
Acepromazine Butorphanol	0.05 mg/kg i.m. or s.c. 0.4 mg/kg i.m. or s.c.	0.05 mg/kg i.m. or s.c. 0.4 mg/kg i.m. or s.c.	0.02–0.05 mg/kg i.m. 0.2–0.4 mg/kg i.m.
Acepromazine Methadone	– 	– 	0.05–0.10 mg/kg i.m 0.1 mg/kg i.m.
Acepromazine Morphine	0.05 mg/kg i.m. or s.c. 0.8 mg/kg i.m. or s.c.	0.05 mg/kg i.m. or s.c. 0.1 mg/kg i.m. or s.c.	–
Acepromazine Oxymorphone	0.03 mg/kg i.m. or s.c. 0.05 mg/kg i.m. or s.c.	0.03 mg/kg i.m. or s.c. 0.05 mg/kg i.m. or s.c.	–
Detomidine Butorphanol	0.04 mg/kg i.m. 0.4 mg/kg i.m.	– 	0.010–0.015 mg/kg i.m. 0.02–0.03 mg/kg i.m.
Romifidine Butorphanol	– 	0.04 mg/kg i.m. 0.4 mg/kg i.m.	0.05 mg/kg i.m. 0.02–0.03 mg/kg i.m.
Xylazine Butorphanol	0.3 mg/kg i.m. 0.4 mg/kg i.m.	0.3 mg/kg i.m. 0.4 mg/kg i.m.	0.5–1.0 mg/kg i.m. 0.02 mg/kg i.m.
Detomidine Methadone	– 	– 	0.010–0.015 mg/kg i.m. 0.1 mg/kg i.m.
Xylazine Methadone	– 	– 	0.5 mg/kg i.m. 0.1 mg/kg i.m.
Acepromazine Butorphanol	– 	– 	0.04–0.06 mg/kg i.m. 0.1–0.2 mg/kg i.m.
Detomidine Acepromazine	– 	– 	0.010–0.015 mg/kg i.m. 0.04–0.06 mg/kg i.m.
Methadone Detomidine	– 	– 	0.05–0.10 mg/kg i.m. 0.010–0.015 mg/kg i.m.

Table 5.10 Sedative/analgesic combinations for the dog, cat and horse. Including an analgesic in preanaesthetic medication results in pre-emptive analgesia (see text).

mg/kg i.v. or i.m.) can be given 2–3 times per day to provide several days analgesia. This may reduce gut motility but does not usually cause impaction. It is also used in the treatment of colic and for postoperative analgesia.

In general, opioids are believed to be more effective for visceral pain than skeletal pain in horses. In addition, in view of the potential for decreased gut motility, they are often withheld from the horse with colic, after a single dose, due to the concern for inducing or exacerbating ileus. There is considerable clinical experience that opioids are an extremely valuable adjunct to management of the horse with skeletal pain, particularly pre- and postoperatively. As in other species, the combination of an opioid and a NSAID provides the most effective analgesia.

Local Analgesia

Local anaesthetics are frequently used to provide analgesia for surgery in locations where suitable nerve blocks can be carried out. These agents also provide excellent postoperative analgesia, particularly when longer-acting drugs (e.g. bupivacaine) are used. They must be used with care after orthopaedic surgery as the horse must retain adequate perception of the injured limb. Lidocaine is not usually used in horses, as it causes tissue oedema. Mepivacaine is the preferred agent as the vehicle is less irritant than other preparations, and so produces less local oedema. After infiltration of local anesthetics, some tissue swelling may result but it is rarely a clinical problem, and does not delay wound healing.

Alpha-2 adrenoceptor agonists

These drugs are commonly used for their visceral analgesic effect in horses. This analgesic effect is partly mediated by a reduction in gut motility, and it is, therefore, essential that a diagnosis and appropriate treatment is concurrent with their use in horses presenting with abdominal pain (see chapter 7).

The alpha-2 adrenoreceptor agonists cause cardiovascular depression as in other species and considerable care in their use is essential in horses likely to require anaesthesia for colic surgery. Nonetheless, used judiciously these are excellent drugs to allow a relatively stress-free colic workup, preoperative preparation and intraoperative analgesia.

Ketamine

This drug is widely used for induction of anaesthesia in horses and also commonly used in incremental doses to supplement volatile agent anaesthesia. It has been shown to reduce MAC in horses (Muir & Sams 1992) and may have a pre-emptive analgesic effect when used during anaesthesia, as in other species (Slingsby 1999).

Adjuncts to pain relief

As with other species, horses respond well to effective support of an injured area so that the damaged tissue is immobilised. Since it is essential that a horse is able to stand up, good support of a fractured limb is also vital in preventing further damage. In addition to this, the horse should be restricted in a small stable as immobility will enhance the effect of analgesics.

The argument that pain relief should not be provided so that the animal does not use the limb and thus damage it further may be more applicable in horses than in smaller species (see chapter 1), as there is no doubt that their sheer bulk and weight can lead to serious damage if excessive stress is placed on a recently repaired limb fracture. However, it is quite unnecessary to withhold analgesics as some protective reflexes are always retained (see chapter 1). It is more important to avoid rendering the horse ataxic through excessive use of analgesics and sedatives. In addition, bandaging and splinting can be used to provide support for the limb. Such support will not only protect the limb but will also enhance analgesia. Such support will not only protect the limb but will also enhance analgesia.

Ruminants

NSAIDs

These agents can be used safely and effectively in domestic and exotic ruminants. They are useful both for controlling postsurgical pain and for other types of both chronic and acute pain. Their relatively long duration of action may make them more useful in clinical practice than opioids (see below).

Opioids

Opioids are effective analgesics in ruminants although most opioids have relatively short durations of action in sheep, because this species metabolises most drugs very rapidly. For example, pethidine (meperidine) is effective for less than 30 minutes in sheep (Nolan et al 1988), although buprenorphine may last for up to 4 hours. Concurrent use of NSAIDs is therefore likely to be particularly beneficial in this species, as is use of alternative routes of drug administration, such as epidural administration. High doses of opioids cause agitation and compulsive chewing behaviour in sheep.

Butorphanol (0.05–0.10 mg/kg i.v.) combined with diazepam (0.05–0.20 mg/kg i.v.) appears particularly useful for sedation of small ruminants, especially those with painful lesions.

Alpha-2 adrenoreceptor agonists

Ruminants have a high density of alpha-2 adrenoreceptors compared to opioid receptors, so alpha-2 agonists (e.g. xylazine) are likely to be more effective analgesics in these species (Nolan et al 1987, Grant et al 1996). Continuous infusion of these agents (e.g. xylazine 0.08–0.10 mg/kg i.m., then 0.03–0.04 mg/kg i.v.) may provide effective, prolonged analgesia (Grant 1999, personal communication) although care must be taken when using these drugs in sheep because of the severe hypoxia that can be produced (see chapter 3).

Pigs

There have been very few clinical trials of analgesic use in pigs, and few drugs are licensed for use in this species. Nevertheless, since pigs are used in surgical research, analgesic use for the control of postsurgical pain has been widespread.

NSAIDs

In the author's experience, carprofen and flunixin can both be used to control postsurgical pain in pigs, and can be administered by intravenous or subcutaneous injection for up to 3 days. Ketoralac has been shown to be effective following major surgery (Andersen et al 1998). Oral NSAIDs (e.g. aspirin, paracetamol) can be used to control mild pain, or chronic mild to moderate pain (e.g. arthritis).

Opioids

Pigs appear relatively insensitive to short-acting opioids such as fentanyl, and relatively high doses (200 µg/kg) are needed to produce significant analgesic effects intraoperatively (Moon et al 1995). Buprenorphine and pethidine have both been shown to be effective using thermal analgesiometry, although pethidine (meperidine) has a short duration of action (as in other species) (Hermansen et al 1986). The dose of buprenorphine used in this experimental study (0.1 mg/kg) is almost certainly higher than that needed to control clinical pain, and in most instances dose rates up to 0.01 mg/kg appear adequate (Table 5.4). Fentanyl patches have been used in pigs with moderate success (Harvey-Clarke et al 2000). Epidural opioids (e.g. diamorphine and fentanyl) can also be used successfully in pigs to control postsurgical pain. Dose rates used have been estimated by extrapolation from man.

Local anaesthetic

As in other species, epidural local anaesthetics can be used in pigs, as can intercostal nerve block. EMLA cream is effective in preventing transient pain associated with blood sampling or injection of the ear veins.

Rabbits and small rodents

NSAIDs

Although there have been few controlled clinical trials of NSAIDs in small mammals, considerable basic data are available concerning likely effective dose rates of these agents in laboratory species (Liles & Flecknell 1992). The duration of action of the more potent NSAIDs such as carprofen and flunixin in rodents and rabbits is uncertain, but clinical experience suggests that a single dose may provide up to 24 hours of analgesia. Clinical experience in the use of flunixin, carprofen, ketoprofen and meloxicam is growing rapidly, and to date, no reports of adverse reactions have been published. Nevertheless, it seems advisable to adopt the same precautions as in dogs and cats. Prolonged use (more than a few days) should be avoided when possible, and preoperative administration of most NSAIDs (with the exception of carprofen) should be avoided because of the potential for renal toxicity should hypotension occur during anaesthesia.

Opioids

As with the NSAIDs, there are few controlled clinical trials, but very extensive amounts of basic data exist that can be used to suggest appropriate dose rates of opioids in rabbits and rodents. One practical problem associated with the use of opioids arises from their relatively short duration of action. This is likely to be a particular problem in small rodents, since they have disproportionately faster rates of drug metabolism than larger species (Morris 1995). For this reason, buprenorphine, which has a prolonged duration of action in most species, is to be preferred in small mammals. Experience of using buprenorphine indicates that dosing at 8–12 hour intervals is effective in controlling most postsurgical pain in rodents and rabbits. Most rodents and rabbits seem to benefit from administration of a single dose of buprenorphine either intraoperatively or immediately postoperatively. If the animal appears to be in pain when reassessed 8 hours later, then a second dose can be administered. This appears to be sufficient for all but the most severe surgical procedures. If pain relief appears inadequate, NSAIDs may be given concurrently with the opioid.

Gastric distension associated with pica has been reported in rats given large doses (0.5 mg/kg s.c.) of buprenorphine, although effects in rats receiving a lower dose (0.05 mg/kg) were minimal (Clark et al 1997). We have frequently observed rats chewing the synthetic sheepskin bedding ('Vetbed', Alfred Cox) in the incubator used for recovery from anaesthesia, but this behaviour is short-lived. In studies carried out in our laboratory, no rats have developed signs of gastric distension, but there are reports of gastric obstruction occurring after the use of buprenorphine (Jacobsen et al 2000). It seems likely that this effect varies with the strain of rat and the anesthetic regimen used. If problems are encountered, then alternative analgesics should be used. If other analgesics are preferred, then morphine, meperidine (pethidine), nalbuphine and butorphanol may all be used, but repeated administration is likely to be needed to provide effective pain relief.

Epidural and intrathecal opioids

An alternative means of providing prolonged analgesia is to administer analgesics by the epidural or intrathecal routes. Opioids given in this way have been shown to have a prolonged effect in man, and to provide effective analgesia. In animals, both clinical and experimental studies have indicated that the technique can be used in a number of species, and it may have practical relevance in the rabbit, since the injection technique is relatively simple (Kero et al 1981).

133

Local anaesthetics

Local anaesthetics can be used to provide analgesia in similar ways to larger species, by infiltration around a surgical field or by use of specific nerve blocks. Some older textbooks mention the potential toxic dangers of local anaesthetics in rats and mice. The dose rates which cause these effects are little different in small mammals from those in dogs and cats, but in very small mammals it is relatively easy to overdose the animal inadvertently. Provided care is taken to calculate the dose accurately, local anaesthetics can be used safely in rodents and rabbits. The effectiveness of agents in providing postsurgical pain relief may be reduced in rodents since the duration of action of agents such as bupivacaine appears to be shorter in rats than in larger species such as dogs, farm animals and human patients (Kitzelshteyn et al 1992).

One use of local anaesthetics that is particularly effective in rabbits is the application of topical agents to provide analgesia for venepuncture or placement of 'over-the-needle' catheters.

Methods of administration

Several practical problems arise when administering analgesics to small mammals. The small muscle mass in these animals, coupled with the relatively high dose rates of some compounds which are needed, can easily lead to tissue damage following intramuscular injection, or to failure of absorption. If possible, this route should be avoided and subcutaneous administration is preferred. Even when using this route, the need for repeated injections of analgesics is both time consuming and may be distressing to the animal, particularly smaller species which require firm physical restraint to enable an injection to be given safely and effectively. Oral dosing can be difficult, although many owners can become adept at administration using a syringe or an infant feeding tube passed into the back of the oral cavity. Provided the animal is eating, then absorption into highly palatable feeds (e.g. doughnuts or spongecake for rats and mice) can be an effective means of drug administration. Use of fruit or meat flavoured jelly can also be effective. The technique was first developed as a means of providing rats with buprenorphine ('Buprenorphine Jell-O,' Pekow 1992; Liles et al 1997), but it soon became apparent that the technique could also be used effectively in mice, and as a means of delivering other agents. To prepare the jelly, commercial flavoured gelatin is reconstituted in half the recommended quantity of water, allowed to cool, then a calculated quantity of drug added. After the jelly sets, it can be cut into cubes of an appropriate weight for feeding. A 200 g rat will eat a 1 ml cube of jelly. The remaining jelly should be carefully labelled and stored in a fridge, taking due note of any legislative requirements concerning storage of controlled substances.

Timing of analgesic administration

Caution is needed when using pre-emptive analgesia in small mammals since injectable anaesthetics are often given as a single, standard dose by intraperitoneal or subcutaneous injection so it is not possible to adjust the dose as anaesthesia is induced. Little information is available concerning the interactions between the commonly used opioids and injectable anaesthetics, so it is advisable to administer opioid analgesics at the end of surgery, when the plane of anaesthesia is lightening, in these smaller species. The NSAID carprofen ('Rimadyl', Pfizer) can be administered safely preoperatively, and when anaesthesia is being induced and maintained using volatile agents, opioids can safely be administered preoperatively. In the author's experience, administration of buprenorphine to rodents prior to anaesthesia with isoflurane results in a 0.25–0.50% reduction in the concentration of anaesthetic required for maintenance.

Additional considerations in postoperative pain relief

Although the use of analgesic drugs remains the most important technique for reducing postoperative pain, the use of these drugs must be integrated into a total scheme for perioperative care. Animals must be provided with a postoperative recovery area appropriate to their particular needs. Remember that allowing a small mammal to recover in the same room as predators (e.g. cats) can be stressful, and can also change their behaviour patterns, masking signs of pain.

Other mammals

There is little published data concerning use of analgesics in non-domestic mammals; however, a large body of clinical experience suggests that most drugs can be used safely and effectively. Suggested dose rates are given in Marx and Roston (1996), and the general principles of extrapolation from the nearest related domestic species, coupled with metabolic scaling (Morris 1995) are usually appropriate.

Birds

Very little information is available concerning the use of analgesics for postoperative pain relief in birds. No clinical trials of their efficacy to control postoperative pain have been undertaken, and only very limited data are available from analgesiometry. However, studies in lame broiler chickens have provided convincing evidence that NSAIDs improve mobility (McGeown et al 1999, Danbury et al 2000). Some studies using analgesiometry suggest that κ agonists (e.g. butorphanol) may be preferable to μ agonists in birds, but given the wide diversity of species involved, this may be a gross oversimplification. Suggestions based on clinical impression include buprenorphine, 0.05 mg/kg i.m., butorphanol, 2–4 mg/kg i.m., or the NSAIDs flunixin (1–10 mg/kg) (Harrison & Harrison 1986), ketoprofen (2 mg/kg) (Wolfensohn & Lloyd 1998), or carprofen (1–4 mg/kg) (A.E. Waterman-Pearson, personal communication).

Reptiles, amphibia and fish

No clinical trials appear to have been undertaken to evaluate analgesic use in these groups of species. Although the antinociceptive effects of some analgesics have been demonstrated in the frog (Stevens et al 1994), these studies all used a form of analgesiometry for assessment. Empirical use of opioids and NSAIDs in reptiles in clinical practice suggests that the drugs can be given to these species without causing obvious adverse effects. Since it is possible that these species may experience pain (see chapter 4), it is advisable, for ethical reasons, to try to provide analgesia in situations that would cause pain in mammals.

References

Adams, H., Mastri, A. and Charron, D. (1977) Morphological effects of subarachnoid methylparaben on rabbit spinal cord. *Pharmacological Research Communications* **9**: 547–551.

Andersen, H.A.E., Fosse, R.T., Kuiper, K. and Nordrehaug, J.E. (1998) Ketorolac (Toradol) as an analgesic in swine following angioplastic and angiographic procedures. *Laboratory Animals* 32(**3**): 307–315.

Bishop, Y. (1998) *The Veterinary Formulary*, 4th edn. Pharmaceutical Press, London.

Bonath, K.H. and Saleh, A.S. (1985) Long term pain treatment in the dog by peridural morphines. *Proceedings of the 2nd International Congress of Veterinary Anesthesia*, pp 160–161 (Abstract).

Borgbjerg, F.M., Svensson, B.A., Frigast, C. et al (1994) Histopathology after repeated intrathecal injections of preservative-free ketamine in the rabbit: a light and electron microscopic examination. *Anesthesia and Analgesia* **79**: 105–111.

Branson, K.R., Ko, J.C.H., Tranquilli, W.J. et al (1993) Duration of analgesia induced by epidurally administered morphine and medetomidine in dogs. *Journal of Veterinary Pharmacology and Therapeutics* **16**: 369–372.

Buggy, D., Hughes, N. and Gardiner, J. (1994) Posterior column sensory impairment during ambulatory extradural analgesia in labour. *British Journal of Anaesthesia* **73**: 540–542.

Cakala, S. (1961) A technique for paravertebral lumbar block in cattle. Cornell Veterinarian **51**: 64–67.

Camann, W.R., Loferski, B.L., Fanciullo, G.J. et al (1992) Does epidural administration of butorphanol offer any clinical advantage over the intravenous route? *Anesthesiology* **76**:216–220.

Capner, C.A., Lascelles, B.D.X., and Waterman-Pearson, A.E. (1999) Current British veterinary attitudes to peri-operative analgesia for dogs. *Veterinary Record* **145**: 95–99.

Cassuto, J., Wallin, G., Hogstrom, S., Faxen, A. and Rimback, G. (1985) Inhibition of postoperative pain by continuous low-dose intravenous infusion of lidocaine. *Anesthesia and Analgesia* **64**: 971–974.

Caulkett, N., Cribb, P.H. and Duke, T. (1993) Xylazine epidural analgesia for cesarean section in cattle. *Canadian Veterinary Journal* **34**: 674–676.

Chapman, C.R. (1985) Psychological factors in postoperative pair. In: Smith, G. and Covino, B.G. (eds) Acute Pain. Butterworths, London, pp 22–41.

Chapman, V. and Dickenson, A.H. (1994) The effect of intrathecal pre- and post-treatment of lignocaine or CNQX on the formalin response of rat dorsal horn neurones. In: *IASP Abstracts, 7th (1993) World Congress on Pain.* IASP Publications, Seattle, p 469.

Chrubasik, J., Vogel, W., Trotschler, H. et al (1987) Continuous-plus-on-demand epidural infusion of buprenorphine versus morphine in postoperative treatment of pain. Postoperative epidural infusion of buprenorphine. *Arzneimittel-Forschung* **37**: 361–363.

Clark, J.A., Myers, P.H., Goelz, M.F., Thigpen, J.E. and Forsythe, D.B. (1997) Pica behaviour associated with buprenorphine administration in the rat. *Laboratory Animal Science* 47(**3**): 300–303.

Clyde, V.L. and Paul-Murphy, J. (1998) Avian analgesia. In: Fowler, M.E. and Miller, R.E. (eds) *Zoo and Wild Animal Medicine, current therapy 4.* W.B. Saunders, Philadelphia, pp 309–314.

Coderre, T.J., Katz, J., Vaccarino, A.L. and Melzack, R. (1993) Contribution of central neuroplasticity to pathological pain: review of clinical and experimental evidence. *Pain* **52**: 259–285.

Cowan, A., Doxey, J.C. and Harry, E.J.R. (1977) The animal pharmacology of buprenorphine, an oripavine analgesic agent. *British Journal of Pharmacology* **60**: 547–554.

Crile, G.W. (1913) The kinetic theory of shock and its prevention through anoci-association (shockless operation). *Lancet* **185**: 7–16.

Csik-Salmon, J., Blais, D., Vaillancourt, D. et al (1996) Utilisation du mélange lidocaine-butorphanol en anesthésie épidurale caudale chez le jument. *Canadian Journal of Veterinary Research* **60**: 288–295.

Cullen, L.K. (1996) Medetomidine sedation in dogs and cats: a review of its pharmacology, antagonism and dose. *British Veterinary Journal* 152(**5**): 519–535.

Dales, B., Bazin, J.E. and Haberer, J.P. (1987) Epidural air bubbles – a cause of incomplete analgesia during epidural anesthesia. *Anesthesia and Analgesia* **66**:679–683.

Danbury, T.C., Weeks, C., Kestin, S.C. and Waterman-Pearson, A.E. (2000) Self-selection of the analgesic drug carprofen by lame broiler chickens. *Veterinary Record* (in press).

Deam, R. and Scott, D. (1993) Neurological damage resulting from extracorporeal shock wave lithotripsy when air is used to locate the epidural space. *Anaesthesia and Intensive Care* **21**: 455–457.

de Castro, G. and Viars, P. (1968) Anesthésie analgesique sequentielle, ou A.A.S. *Archives of Medicine* **23**: 170–176.

de Leon-Casasola, O. and Lema, M. (1994) Epidural bupivacaine/sufentanil therapy for postoperative pain control in patients tolerant to opioid and unresponsive to epidural bupivacaine/morphine. *Anesthesiology* **80**: 303–309.

Dickenson, A.H. and Sullivan, A.F. (1987) Subcutaneous formalin-induced activity of dorsal horn neurons in the rat: differential response to an intrathecal opiate administration pre- or post-formalin. *Pain* **30**: 349–360.

Dickenson, A., Sullivan, A. and McQuay, H. (1990) Intrathecal etorphine, fentanyl and buprenorphine on spinal nociceptive neurones in the rat. *Pain* **42**: 227–234.

Dodman, N.H., Clark, G.H., Court, M.H. et al (1992) Epidural opioid administration for postoperative pain relief in the dog. In: Short, C.E. and Van Poznack, A. (eds) *Animal Pain.* Churchill Livingstone, New York, pp 274–277.

Doherty, T.J. and Frazier, D.L. (1998) Effect of intravenous lidocaine on halothane minimum alveolar concentrations in ponies. *Equine Veterinary Journal* **30**: 329–334.

Doherty, T.J., Geiser, D.R. and Rohrbach, B.W. (1997) Effect of high volume epidural morphine, ketamine and butorphanol on halothane minimum alveolar concentration in ponies. *Equine Veterinary Journal* **29**: 370–373.

Dolan, S. and Nolan, A. (1999) N-methyl D-aspartate induced mechanical allodynia is blocked by nitric oxide synthase and cyclooxygenase-2 inhibitors. *Neuroreport* **10**: 449–452.

Drenger, B. and Magora, F. (1989) Urodynamic studies after intrathecal fentanyl and buprenoprhine in the dog. *Anesthesia and Analgesia* **69**: 348–353.

Drenger, B., Magora, F., Evron, S. et al (1986) The action of intrathecal morphine and methadone on the lower urinary tract in the dog. *Journal of Urology* **135**: 852–855.

Dum, J.E. and Herz, A.L. (1981) In vivo receptor binding of the opiate partial agonist, buprenorphine, correlated with its agonistic and antagonistic actions. *British Journal of Pharmacology* **74**: 627–633.

Durant, P.A.C. and Yaksh, T.L. (1986) Distribution in cerebrospinal fluid, blood, and lymph of epidurally injected morphine and inulin in dogs. *Anesthesia and Analgesia* **65**: 583–592.

Eisenach, J.C., Dewan, D.M., Rose, J.C. et al (1987) Epidural clonidine produces antinociception, but not hypotension, in sheep. *Anesthesiology* **66**: 496–501.

Evron, S., Samueloff, A., Simon, A. et al (1985) Urinary function during epidural analgesia with methadone and morphine in post-cesarean section patients. *Pain* **23**: 135–44.

Farquharson, J. (1940) Paravertebral lumbar anesthetic in the bovine species. *Journal of the American Veterinary Medical Association* **97**: 54–57.

Feldman, H. and Covino, B. (1988) Comparative motor-blocking effects of bupivacaine and ropivacaine, a new amino amide local anesthetic, in the rat and dog. *Anesthesia and Analgesia* **67**: 1047–1052.

Feldman, H.S., Dvoskin, S., Arthur, G.R. et al (1996) Antinociceptive and motor-blocking efficacy of ropivacaine and bupivacaine after epidural administration in the dog. *Regional Anesthesia* **21**: 318–326.

Fischer, R., Lubenow, T., Liceaga, A. et al (1988) Comparison of continuous epidural infusion of fentanyl-bupivacaine and morphine-bupivacaine in management of postoperative pain. *Anesthesia and Analgesia* **67**: 559–563.

Flecknell, P.A. (1996) *Laboratory Animal Anaesthesia*, 2nd edn. Academic Press, London

Flecknell, P.A., Liles, J.H. and Wootton, R. (1989) Reversal of fentanyl/fluanisone neuroleptanalgesia in the rabbit using mixed agonist/antagonist opioids. *Laboratory Animals* **23**: 147–155.

Flecknell, P.A., Liles, J.H. and Williamson, H.A. (1990a) The use of lignocaine-prilocaine local anaesthetic cream for pain-free venepuncture in laboratory animals. *Laboratory Animals* **24**: 142–146.

Flecknell, P.A., Kirk, A.J.B., Fox, C.E. and Dark, J.H. (1990b) Long-term anaesthesia with propofol and alfentanil in the dog and its partial reversal with nalbuphine. *Journal of the Association of Veterinary Anaesthetists* **17**: 11–16.

Ford, D. and Raj, P. (1987) Peripheral neurotoxicity of 2-chloroprocaine and bisulfite in the cat. *Anesthesia and Analgesia* **66**: 719–22.

Gallivan, S.T., Johnston, S.J., Broadstone, R. et al (1999) The safety of epidurally administered ketorolac in dogs. *Veterinary Surgery* **28**: 393 (Abstract).

Gaumann, D.M., Brunet, P.C. and Jirounek, P. (1992) Clonidine enhances the effects of lidocaine on C-fiber action potential. *Anesthesia and Analgesia* **74**: 719–725.

Gilroy, B.A. (1982) Effect of intercostal nerve blocks on post-thoracotomy ventilation and oxygenation in the canine. *Journal of Veterinary Care* **6**: 1–9.

Golder, F.J., Pascoe, P.J., Binley, C.S., et al (1998) The effect of epidural morphine on the minimum alveolar concentration of isoflurane in cats. *Journal of Veterinary Anaesthesia* **25**: 52–56.

Gomez, S.I.A., Rossi, R., Santos, M. et al (1998) Epidural injection of ketamine for perineal analgesia in the horse. *Veterinary Surgery* **27**: 384–391.

Goodrich, L.R., Nixon, A.J., Fubini, S.L. et al (1999) Efficacy of epidurally administered morphine and detomidine in decreasing postoperative hind limb lameness in horses following bilateral stifle arthroscopy. *Veterinary Surgery* **28**: 393 (Abstract).

Grant, C., Upton, R.N. and Kuchel, T.R. (1996) An assessment of the efficacy of intramuscular analgesics for acute pain in the sheep. *Australian Veterinary Journal* **25**: 129–132.

Grubb, T.L., Riebold, T.W. and Huber, M.J. (1991) Comparison of lidocaine, xylazine, and xylazine/lidocaine for equine caudal epidural anaesthesia. *Journal of Veterinary Anaesthesia* **3**(Suppl.): 369 (abstract).

Grubb, T.L., Riebold, T.W. and Huber, M.J. (1993) Evaluation of lidocaine, xylazine, and a combination of lidocaine and xylazine for epidural analgesia in llamas. *Journal of the American Veterinary Medical Association* **203**: 1441–1444.

Hall, L.W. and Clark, K.W. (1991) *Veterinary Anaesthesia* 8th edn. Baillière Tindall, London.

Harrison, G.J. and Harrison, L.R. (1986) *Clinical Avian Medicine and Surgery*. W.B. Saunders, Philadelphia.

Harvey-Clarke, C.J., Gilespie, K. and Riggs, K.W. (2000) Transdermal fentanyl compared to parenteral buprenorphine in post-surgical pain in swine: a case study. *Laboratory Animals* (in press).

Heath, R.B., Broadstone, R.V., Wright, M. et al (1985) Bupivacaine and mepivacaine lumbosacral epidural analgesia in dogs. *Proceedings of the 2nd International Congress of Veterinary Anesthesia*, pp 162 163 (Abstract).

Hermansen, K., Pedersen, L.E. and Olesen, H.O. (1986) The analgesic effect of buprenorphine, etorphine and pethidine in the pig: a randomized double blind cross-over study. *Acta Pharmacologica et Toxicologica* **59**: 27–35.

Herperger, L.J. (1998) Postoperative urinary retention in a dog following morphine with bupivacaine epidural analgesia. *Canadian Veterinary Journal* **39**: 650–652.

Hirota, K. and Lambert, D.G. (1996) Ketamine: its mechanism(s) of action and unusual clinical uses. *British Journal of Anaesthesia* **77**: 441–444.

Hu, C., Flecknell, P.A. and Liles, J.H. (1992). Fentanyl and medetomidine anaesthesia in the rat and its reversal using atipamazole and either nalbuphine or butorphanol. *Laboratory Animals* **26**: 15–22.

Inagaki, Y. and Kuzukawa, A. (1997) Effects of epidural and intravenous buprenorphine on halothane minimum alveolar anesthetic concentration and hemodynamic responses. *Anesthesia and Analgesia* **84**: 100–105.

Inagaki, Y., Mashimo, T. and Yoshiya, I. (1996) Mode and site of analgesic action of epidural buprenorphine in humans. *Anesthesia and Analgesia* **83**: 530–536.

Islas, J., Astorga, J. and Laredo, M. (1985) Epidural ketamine for control of postoperative pain. *Anesthesia and Analgesia* **64**: 1161–1162.

Jacobsen, C. (2000) Adverse effects on growth rate in rats caused by buprenorphine administration. *Laboratory Animals* (in press).

Jaffe, R. and Rowe, M. (1996) A comparison of the local anesthetic effects of meperidine, fentanyl, and sufentanil on dorsal root axons. *Anesthesia and Analgesia* **83**: 776–781.

Johnson, C.B. and Taylor, P.M. (1997) Effects of alfentanil on the equine electroencephalogram during anaesthesia with halothane in oxygen. *Research in Veterinary Science* **62**: 159–163.

Junega, M., Kargas, G.A., Miller, D.L. et al (1995) Comparison of epidural catheter induced paresthesia in parturients. *Regional Anaesthesia* **20** (Suppl.): 152 (Abstract).

Junega, M., Kargas, G.A., Miller, D.L. et al (1996) Incidence of epidural vein cannulation in parturients with three different epidiural catheters. *Regional Anaesthesia* **21** (Suppl.): 4 (Abstract).

Kamerling, S.G., DeQuick, D.J., Weckman, T.J. and Tobin, T. (1985) Dose-related effects of fentanyl on autonomic and behavioral responses in performance horses. *General Pharmacology* **16**: 253–258.

Kawana, Y., Sato, H., Shimada, H. et al (1987) Epidural ketamine for postoperative pain relief after gynecologic operations: a double-blind study and comparison with epidural morphine. *Anesthesia and Analgesia* **66**: 735–738.

Keegan, R.D., Greene, S.A. and Weil, A.B. (1995) Cardiovascular effects of epidurally administered morphine and a xylazine-morphine combination in isoflurane-anesthetized dogs. *American Journal of Veterinary Research* **56**: 496–500.

Kelawala, N.H., Amresh, K., Chaudary, S. et al (1996) Effects of epidural xylazine with diazepam premedication in dogs. *Indian Veterinary Journal* **73**: 552–557.

Kero, P., Thomasson, B. and Soppi, A.M. (1981) Spinal anaesthesia in the rabbit. *Laboratory Animals* **15**: 347–348.

King, J.N. and Gerring, E.L. (1989) Antagonism of endotoxin induced disruption of equine bowel motility by flunixin and phenylbutazone. *Equine Veterinary Journal* **7** (Suppl.): 38–42.

Kitzelshteyn, G., Bairamian, M., Inchiosa, M.A. and Chase, J.E. (1992) Enhancement of bupivacaine sensory blockade of rat sciatic nerve by combination with phenol. *Anesthesia and Analgesia* **74**: 499–502.

Ko, J.C.H., Thurmon, J.C., Benson, J.G. et al (1992) Evaluation of analgesia induced by epidural injection of detomidine or xylazine in swine. *Journal of Veterinary Anaesthesia* **19**: 56–60.

Kristensen, J.D., Svensson, B. and Gordh, T.J. (1992) The NMDA-receptor antagonist CPP abolishes neurogenic 'wind-up pain' after intrathecal administration in humans. *Pain* **51**: 249–253.

Kristensen, J.D., Karlsten, R., Gordh, T. et al (1994) The NMDA antagonist 3-(2-carboxypiperazin-4-yl)propyl-1-phosphonic acid (CPP) has antinociceptive effect after intrathecal injection in the rat. *Pain* **56**: 59–67.

Lascelles, B.D.X., Butterworth, S.J. and Waterman, A.E. (1994) Postoperative analgesic and sedative effects of carprofen and pethidine in dogs. *Veterinary Record* **134**: 187–191.

Lascelles, B.D.X., Waterman, A.E., Cripps, P.J., Livingston, A. and Henderson, G. (1995) Central sensitization as a result of surgical pain: investigation of the pre-emptive value of pethidine for ovariohysterectomy in the rat. *Pain* **62**: 201–212.

Lascelles, B.D.X., Cripps, P.J., Jones, A. and Waterman-Pearson, A.E. (1997) Post-operative central hypersensitivity and pain: the pre-emptive value of pethidine for ovariohysterectomy. *Pain* 73(**3**): 461–471.

Lascelles, B.D.X., Cripps, P.J., Jones, A. and Waterman-Pearson, A.E. (1998) Efficacy and kinetics of carprofen, administered preoperatively or postoperatively, for the prevention of pain in dogs undergoing ovariohysterectomy. *Veterinary Surgery* **27**: 568–582.

Latasch, L., Probst, S. and Dudziak, R. (1984) Reversal by nalbuphine of respiratory depression caused by fentanyl. *Anesthesia and Analgesia* **63**: 814–816.

Lebeaux, M.I. (1973) Experimental epidural anaesthesia in the dog with lignocaine and bupivacaine. *British Journal of Anaesthesia* **45**: 549–555.

Liles, J.H. and Flecknell, P.A. (1992) The use of non-steroidal anti-inflammatory drugs for the relief of pain in laboratory rodents and rabbits. *Laboratory Animals* **26**: 241–255.

Liles, J.H., Flecknell, P.A., Roughan, J.A. and Cruz-Madorran, I. (1997) Influence of oral buprenorphine, oral naltrexone or morphine on the effects of laparotomy in the rat. *Laboratory Animals* **32**: 149–161.

Loper, K.A., Ready, L.B., Downey, M. et al (1990) Epidural and intravenous fentanyl infusion are clinically equivalent after knee surgery. *Anesthesia and Analgesia* **70**: 72–75.

McCrackin, M.A., Harvey, R.C., Sackman, J.E., McLean, R.A. and Paddleford, R.R. (1994) Butorphanol tartrate for partial reversal of oxymorphone-induced postoperative respiratory depression in the dog. *Veterinary Surgery* **23**: 67–74.

McGeown, D., Danbury T.C., Waterman-Pearson, A.E. and Kestin, S.C. (1999) Effect of carprofen on lameness in broiler chickens. *Veterinary Record* **144**: 668–671.

Malley, D. (1999) Reptiles. In: Seynour, C. and Gleed, R. (eds) Manual of Small Animal Anaesthesia and Analgesia. BSAVA, Cheltenham, pp 271–282.

Malmberg, A.B. and Yaksh, T.L. (1993) Pharmacology of the spinal action of ketorolac, morphine, ST-91, U50488H, and L-PIA on the formalin test and an isobolographic analysis of the NSAID interaction. *Anesthesiology* **79**: 270–281.

Mama, K.R., Pascoe, P.J. and Steffey, E.P. (1992) Evaluation of the interaction of mu and kappa opioid agonists on locomotor behaviour in the horse. *Canadian Journal of Veterinary Research* **57**: 106–109.

Marx, K.L. and Roston, M.A. (1996) *The Exotic Animal Drug Compendium*. Veterinary Learning Systems, New Jersey, USA.

Mather, L.G. (1983) Pharmacokinetic and pharmacodynamic factors influencing the choice, dose and route of administration of opiates for acute pain. *Clinics in Anaesthesiology* **1**: 17–40.

Mazoit, J.X., Lambert, C. and Berdeauz, A. (1988) Pharmacokinetics of bupivacaine after short and prolonged infusions in conscious dogs. *Anesthesia and Analgesia* **67**: 961–966.

Miwa, Y., Yonemura, E. and Fukushima, K. (1996) Epidural administered buprenorphine in the perioperative period. *Canadian Journal of Anaesthesia* **43**: 907–913.

Mollenholt, P., Post, C., Paulsson, I. et al (1990) Intrathecal and epidural somatostatin in rats: can antinociception, motor effects and neurotoxicity be separated? *Pain* **43**: 363–370.

Molloy, R.E. and Benzon, H.T. (1996) The current status of epidural steroids. *Current Reviews of Pain* **1**: 61–69.

Monasky, M.S., Zinsmeister, A.R., Stevens, C.W. et al (1990) Interaction of intrathecal morphine and ST-91 on antinociception in the rat: dose-response analysis, antagonism and clearance. *Journal of Pharmacology and Experimental Therapeutics* **254**: 383–392.

Moon, P.F., Scarlett, J.M., Ludders, J.W., Conway T.A. and Lamb, S.V. (1995) Effect of fentanyl on the medium alveolar concentration of isoflurane in swine. *Anesthesiology* **83**: 535–542.

Moon, P. and Suter, C.M. (1993) Paravertebral thoracolumbar anesthesia in ten horses. Equine Veterinary Journal **25**: 304–308.

Morris, T.H. (1995) Antibiotic therapeutics in laboratory animals. *Laboratory Animals* **29**: 16–36.

Muir, W.W. III and Sams, R. (1992) Effects of ketamine infusion on halothane minimum alveolar concentration in horses. *American Journal of Veterinary Research* **53**: 1802–1806.

Naguib, M., Adu-Gyamfi, Y., Absood, G. et al (1986) Epidural ketamine for postoperative analgesia. *Canadian Anaesthesia Society Journal* **33**: 16–21.

Nemirovsky, A. and Niv, D. (1996) Cholinergic mechanisms and antinociception. *Current Reviews of Pain* **1**: 10–22.

Nolan, A., Livingston, A. and Waterman, A. (1987) Antinociceptive actions of intravenous α2-adrenoceptor agonists in sheep. *Journal of Veterinary Pharmacology and Therapeutics* **10**: 202–209.

Nolan, A., Waterman, A.E. and Livingston, A. (1988) The correlation of the thermal and mechanical antinociceptive activity of pethidine hydrochloride with plasma concentrations of the drug in sheep. *Journal of Veterinary Pharmacology and Therapeutics* **11**: 94–102.

Olek, A. and Edwards, C. (1980) Effects of anesthetic treatment on motor neuron death in xenopus. *Brain Research* **191**: 483–488.

Pascoe, P.J. (1993) Analgesia after lateral thoracotomy in dogs. Epidural morphine vs. intercostal bupivacaine. *Veterinary Surgery* 22(2): 141–147.

Pascoe, P.J. and Taylor, P.M. (1997) Is opioid-induced locomotor activity in horses dopamine mediated? *Proceedings of the 6th International Congress on Veterinary Anaesthesia*, p 131.

Peat, S., Bras, P. and Hanna, M. (1989) A double-blind comparison of epidural ketamine and diamorphine for postoperative analgesia. *Anaesthesia* **44**: 555–558.

Pekow, C. (1992) Buprenorphine Jell-O recipe for rodent analgesia. *Synapse* 25(3): 35–36.

Popilskis, S., Kohn, D., Sanchez, J.A. et al (1991) Epidural vs. intramuscular oxymorphone analgesia after thoracotomy in dogs. *Veterinary Surgery* **20**: 462–467.

Popilskis, S., Kohn, D.F., Laurent, L. et al (1993) Efficacy of epidural morphine versus intravenous morphine for post-thoracotomy pain in dogs. *Journal of Veterinary Anaesthesia* **20**: 21–25.

Quandt, J.E., Raffe, M.R. and Robinson, E.P. (1994) Butorphanol does not reduce the minimum alveolar concentration of halothane in dogs. *Veterinary Surgery* **23**: 156–159.

Rane, K., Segerdahl, M., Goiny, M. et al (1998) Intrathecal adenosine administration: a phase 1 clinical safety study in healthy volunteers, with additional evaluation of its influence on sensory thresholds and experimental pain. *Anesthesiology* **89**: 1108–1115.

Rawal, N., Nuutinen, L., Raj, P. et al (1991) Behavioral and histopathologic effects following intrathecal administration of butorphanol, sufentanil, and nalbuphine in sheep. *Anesthesiology* **75**: 1025–1034.

Rector, E., Kramer, S., Kietzmann, M. et al (1998) Analgesic effect of xylazine, injected systemically or epidurally into dogs anaesthetized with isoflurane. *Berliner und Munchener Tierarztliche Wochenschrift* **111**: 438–451.

Richmond, C.E., Bromley, L.M. and Woolf, C.J. (1993) Pre-operative morphine pre-empts post-operative pain. *Lancet* **342**: 73–75.

Robinson, E.P., Moncada-Suarez, J.R. and Felice, L. (1994) Epidural morphine analgesia in horses. *Veterinary Surgery* **23**: 78 (Abstract).

Rolbin, S.H., Hew, E. and Ogilvie, G. (1987) A comparison of two types of epidural catheters. *Canadian Journal of Anaesthesia* **34**: 459–461.

Rosseel, M., Van Den Broek, W.G.M., Boer, E.C. et al (1988) Epidural sufentanil for intra- and postoperative analgesia in thoracic surgery: a comparative study with intravenous sufentanil. *Acta Anaesthesiologica Scandinavica* **32**: 193–198.

Sabbe, M.B., Penning, J.P., Ozaki, G.T. et al (1994) Spinal and systemic action of the alpha 2 receptor agonist dexmedetomidine in dogs. Antinociception and carbon dioxide response. *Anesthesiology* **80**: 1057–1072.

Sammarco, J.L., Conzemius, M.G., Perkowski, S.Z., Weinstein, M.J., Gregor, T.P. and Smith, G.K. (1996) Post-operative analgesia for stifle surgery: a comparison of intra-articular bupivacaine, morphine, or saline. *Veterinary Surgery* **25**: 59–69.

Sethna, N. and Berde, C. (1993) Venous air embolism during identification of the epidural space in children. *Anesthesia and Analgesia* **76**: 925–927.

Sjöström, S., Hartvig, D. and Tamsen, A. (1988) Patient-controlled analgesia with extradural morphine or pethidine. *British Journal of Anaesthesia* **60**: 358–366.

Skarda, R.T. (1996a) Local and regional anesthetic and analgesic techniques: horses. In: Thurmon, J.C., Tranquilli, W.J. and Benson, G.J. (eds) *Lumb and Jones Veterinary Anesthesia*, 3rd edn. Williams and Wilkins, Baltimore, pp 448–478.

Skarda, R.T. (1996b) Local and regional anesthetic and analgesic techniques: ruminants and swine. In: Thurmon, J.C., Tranquilli, W.J. and Benson, G.J. (eds) *Lumb and Jones Veterinary Anesthesia*, 3rd edn. Williams and Wilkins, Baltimore, pp 499–514.

Skarda, R.T. and Muir, W.W. III (1994) Caudal analgesia induced by epidural or subarachnoid administration of detomidine hydrochloride solution in mares. *American Journal of Veterinary Research* **55**: 670–680.

Skarda, R.T. and Muir, W.W. III (1996) Comparison of antinociceptive, cardiovascular, and respiratory effects, head ptosis, and position of pelvic limbs in mares after caudal epidural administration of xylazine and detomidine hydrochloride. *American Journal of Veterinary Research* **57**: 1338–1345.

Skarda, R.T., St Jean G.S. and Muir, W.W. (1990) Influence of tolazoline on caudal epidural administration of xylazine in cattle. *American Journal of Veterinary Research* **51**: 556–560.

Slingsby, L.S. and Waterman-Pearson, A.E. (1996) Postoperative analgesia in the cat: a comparison of pethidine, buprenorphine, ketoprofen and carprofen. *Journal of Veterinary Anesthesia* 24: 43.

Slingsby, L.S. and Waterman-Pearson, A.E. (1998) Comparison of pethidine, buprenorphine and ketoprofen for postoperative analgesia after ovariohysterectomy in the cat. *Veterinary Record* **143**: 185–189.

Slingsby, L.S. (1999) Studies on perioperative analgesia in the dog, cat and rat. PhD thesis. University of Bristol, Bristol, pp 147–182.

Stanway, G.W., Brodbelt, D.C. and Taylor, P.M. (1996) A comparison of preoperative morphine and buprenorphine in cats. *Journal of Veterinary Anaesthesia* 23: 78.

Stevens, R., Mikat-Stevens, M., Van Clief, M. et al (1989) Deliberate epidural air injection in dogs: a radiographic study. *Regional Anesthesia* **14**: 180–182.

Stevens, C.W., Klopp, A.J, Facello, J.A. (1994) Analgesic potency of mu and kappa opioids after systemic administration in amphibians 1. *Journal of Pharmacology and Experimental Therapeutics* 269(**3**): 1086–1093.

Stevens, R.A., Petty, R.H., Hill, H.F. et al (1993) Redistribution of sufentanil to cerebrospinal fluid and systemic circulation after epidural administration in dogs. *Anesthesia and Analgesia* **76**: 323–327.

Sysel, A.M., Pleasant, R.S., Jacobson, J.D. et al (1996) Efficacy of an epidural combination of morphine and detomidine in alleviating experimentally induced hindlimb lameness in horses. *Veterinary Surgery* **25**: 511–518.

Tanelian, D.L. and MacIver, M.B. (1991) Analgesic concentrations of lidocaine suppress tonic A-delta and C fiber discharges produced by acute injury. *Anesthesiology* **74**: 934–936.

Taylor, P.M. and Clarke, K.W. (1999) *Handbook of Equine Anesthesia.* Baillière Tindall, London pp 27–28.

Thompson, S.E. and Johnson, J.M. (1991) Analgesia in dogs after intercostal thoracotomy. A comparison of morphine, selective intercostal nerve block, and interpleural regional analgesia with bupivacaine. *Veterinary Surgery* 20(1): 73–77.

Thurmon, J.C., Tranquilli, W.J. and Benson, G.J. (1996) *Lumb and Jones Veterinary Anaesthesia,* 3rd edn. Williams and Wilkins, Baltimore.

Thurston, C.L., Culhane, E.S., Suberg, S.N. et al (1988) Antinociception vs motor effects of intrathecal vasopressin as measured by four pain tests. *Brain Research* **463**: 1–11.

Tobin, T. (1978) Pharmacology review: Narcotic analgesics and opiate receptors in the horse. *Journal of Equine Medicine and Surgery* **2**: 397–399.

Torda, T.A. and Pybus, D.A. (1982) Comparison of four narcotic analgesics for extradural analgesia. *British Journal of Anaesthesia* **54**: 291–295.

Troncy, E., Cuvelliez, S. and Blais, D. (1996) Evaluation of analgesia and cardiorespiratory effects of epidurally administered butorphanol in isoflurane-anesthetized dogs. *American Journal of Veterinary Research* **57**: 1478–1482.

Tung, A.S. and Yaksh, T.L. (1982) The antinociceptive effects of epidural opiates in the cat: Studies on the pharmacology and the effects of lipophilicity in spinal analgesia. *Pain* **12**: 343–356.

Tverskoy, M., Oz, Y., Iakson, A., Finger, J., Bradley E.L. Jr, Kissin, I. (1994) Pre-emptive effect of fentanyl and ketamine on postoperative pain and wound hyperalgesia. *Anesthesia and Analgesia* **78**: 205–209.

Valverde, A., Little, C.B., Dyson, D.H. et al (1990) Use of epidural morphine to relieve pain in a horse. *Canadian Veterinary Journal* **31**: 211–212.

Valverde, A., Dyson, D.H., McDonell, W.N. (1989) Epidural morphine reduces halothane MAC in the dog. *Canadian Journal Anaesthesia* **36**: 629–632.

Valverde, A., Dyson, D.H., Cockshutt, J.R. et al (1991) Comparison of the hemodynamic effects of halothane alone and halothane combined with epidurally administered morphine for anesthesia in ventilated dogs. *American Journal of Veterinary Research* **52**: 505–509.

Vesal, N., Cribb, P. and Frketic, M. (1996) Postoperative analgesic and cardiopulmonary effects in dogs of oxymorphone administered epidurally and intramuscularly, and medetomidine administered epidurally: a comparative clinical study. *Veterinary Surgery* **25**: 361–369.

Walmsley, P. bandaging horses

Wang, B.C., Li, D., Hiller, J.M. et al (1992) Lumbar subarachnoid ethylene diamine tetraacetate induces hindlimb tetanic contractions in rats: prevention by $CaCl_2$ pretreatment; observation of spinal nerve root degeneration. *Anesthesia and Analgesia* **75**: 895–899.

Wang, C., Chakrabarti, M.K. and Whitwam, J.G. (1993) Specific enhancement by fentanyl of the effects of intrathecal bupivacaine on nociceptive afferent but not sympathetic efferent pathways in dogs. *Anesthesiology* **79**: 766–733.

Wang, B.C., Li, D., Budzilovich, G. et al (1994) Antinociception without motor blockade after subarachnoid administration of S-(+)ibuprofen in rats. *Life Science* **54**: 15–720.

Wang, B.C., Li, D., Hiller, J.M. et al (1995) The antinociceptive effect of S–(+)-ibuprofen in rabbits: epidural versus intravenous administration. *Anesthesia and Analgesia* **80**: 92–96.

Waterman, A.E. and Kalthum, W. (1989) The absorption and distribution of subcutaneously administered pethidine in the dog. *Journal of the Association of Veterinary Anaesthetists* **16**: 51–52.

Watkins, L., Kinscheck, I. and Mayer, D. (1985) Potentiation of morphine analgesia by the cholecystokinin antagonist proglumide. *Brain Research* **327**: 169–180.

Welsh, E.M., Nolan, A.M. and Reid, J. (1997) Beneficial effects of administering carprofen before surgery in dogs. *Veterinary Record* **141**: 251–253.

Wolfensohn, S. and Lloyd, M. (1998) *Handbook of Laboratory Animal Management and Welfare*, 2nd edn. Oxford University Press, Oxford.

Wong, C., Liaw, W., Tung, C. et al (1996) Ketamine potentiates analgesic effect of morphine in postoperative epidural pain control. *Regional Anesthesia* **21**: 534–541.

Wong, C., Cherng, C. and Tung, C. (1998) Intrathecal administration of excitatory amino acid receptor antagonists or nitric oxide synthase inhibitor reduced autotomy behaviour in rats. *Anesthesia and Analgesia* **87**: 605–608.

Woolf, C.J. and Wiesenfeld-Hallin, Z. (1985) The systemic administration of local anaesthetics produces a selective depression of C-afferent fibre evoked activity in the spinal cord. *Pain* **23**: 361–374.

Woolf, C.J. and Wall, P.D. (1986) Morphine-sensitive and morphine-insensitive actions of C-fibre input on the rat spinal cord. *Neuroscience Letters* **64**: 221–225.

Yaksh, T. (1996) Epidural ketamine: a useful, mechanistically novel adjuvant for epidural morphine? *Regional Anesthesia* **21**: 508–513.

Yang, J. (1994) Intrathecal administration of oxytocin induces analgesia in low back pain involving the endogenous opiate peptide system. *Spine* **19**: 867–871.

Zaric, D., Nydahl, P.A., Phillipson, L. et al (1996) The effect of continuous lumbar epidural infusion of ropivacaine (0.1%, 0.2%, and 0.3%) and 0.25% bupivacaine on sensory and motor block in volunteers. *Regional Anesthesia* **21**: 14–25.

CHRONIC PAIN IN ANIMALS

6

J.C. Brearley, M.J. Brearley

Introduction

The clinical diagnosis and treatment of chronic pain in companion animals presents a multitude of problems. Not the least of these is the inability of animals to verbalise that 'something hurts'; this transfers the responsibility onto the owner and clinician to observe behaviours that 'suggest' pain. Medical physicians treat their patients' reported perception of pain, but in veterinary medicine it is the dysfunction associated with what humans term pain that is treated. Our perception of this dysfunction is coloured by the personal experience of the keeper or the veterinary surgeon's own observation (see chapter 4).

Chronic or long-term subclinical pain in farm animals may manifest itself as a reduction in milk production or as a decreased rate of growth. These quantifiable output factors are generally not applicable when considering dogs, cats, horses or other mammals. A not uncommon clinical scenario is the aged overweight Labrador that hobbles stiffly after its owner on walks 'obviously in pain' but at mealtime, its appetite is still excellent and the dog 'appears' happy with a good quality of life. Thus, the diagnosis of 'chronic pain' may depend more upon the circumstances of the animal itself than the underlying pathology.

In some situations the diagnosis of chronic pain may be made retrospectively. An owner may report that surgical excision of a tumour has resulted in the dog behaving like a juvenile again after months or years of apparent senescence. From this it may be presumed that the tumour had been causing the dog progressive incapacity for some time and this in part may have been caused by chronic pain.

Chronic pain in companion animals may often be a sequel to a diverse range of underlying problems, also chronic in nature, from osteoarthritis to dental disease to neoplasia. Whilst pain relief is desirable for its own merits, treatment of the underlying cause or compounding factors may be more important in the long term than mere palliation of the secondary problem of chronic pain.

Definition and assessment of chronic pain

The clinical entity of acute pain has been relatively easy to define as a sustained episode of pain which has a relatively short time course. However, the concept of 'chronic pain' was more difficult. The term 'chronic' usually related to the time course rather than to the nature of the pain, and ease of pain control may also be involved in the definition. Pain which cannot be controlled by any means is termed 'intractable'. However, in veterinary medicine, it is often the attending clinician who is responsible for implementing inadequate pain control methods, leading to chronicity, rather than truly intractable pain. It is also important to remember as veterinarians we have the ultimate means for the control of intractable pain, namely euthanasia.

Chronic pain may range from prolonged, continuous and mild to intermittent but severe over an extended time. It may vary in intensity, and bouts of pain may vary in their duration. It is generally accepted that chronic pain has no survival advantage and thus may be termed 'pathological'. This confusion/dilemma of what is classified as chronic pain certainly raises problems when treatment regimens are considered.

Until relatively recently a general theory explained both acute and chronic pain syndromes. This applied the concept of a simple unitary pathway with the noxious event stimulating peripheral receptors which in turn transmitted the information via afferent nerves to the spinal cord and thus to the thalamus via the spinothalamic tracts (see chapter 2). From the thalamus, the information is relayed to other parts of the brain and the appropriate behaviour elicited. Acute pain resulted from a short period of stimulation whereas a prolonged event produced chronic pain.

However, it is now accepted that that this view is too simplistic. Scientific research has proposed and confirmed much about the plasticity of the nervous system and the regulation of neuronal responsiveness which comes into play, particularly with sustained noxious stimuli (see chapter 2). In man, the perception of pain depends on previous experience, present circumstances and surroundings and future projections. The memory of a previously painful experience and the fear of pain in the future may heighten the perception of a present painful event. For further discussion of this see Craig (1994) and Weisenberg (1994).

Recognition of chronic pain

The characteristics of acute and chronic pain in people are given in Table 6.1. Whether these apply directly to animals cannot be answered at present but many will be recognisable to a veterinarian caring for animals in pain. The role of anticipation cannot be easily demonstrated in pet animals. Nevertheless, anecdotally, dogs and cats often show no fear on their initial visit to the veterinary surgery but after a painful experience in these unfamiliar surroundings, there is often a tremendous resistance on their part to re-enter the premises. More objectively, animals show similar motor behaviour patterns and physiological changes to humans when they are exposed to similar noxious stimuli. Unfortunately, most of the experimental methods of assessing pain in animals use acute stimuli and are not applicable to chronic conditions. There are several

Acute pain	Chronic pain
Increased heart rate	Sleep disturbance
Increased stroke volume	Irritability/aggression
Increased blood pressure	Appetite depression
Pupillary dilation	Constipation
Sweating	Mental depression, including immobility
Increased respiratory rate	Lowered pain threshold
Restlessness	Social withdrawal
Avoidance behaviour	Abnormal illness behaviour
Anxiety state	Masked depression

Table 6.1 A comparison of the several 'signs' of pain (after Sternbach 1981).

experimental animal models of chronic tissue injury (Ren & Dubner 1999), e.g. carrageenan foot-pad injections (Iadarola et al 1988), experimentally induced arthritis (De Castro Costa et al 1981, Colpaert 1987) and of neurogenic models of persistent pain, e.g. neuronal ligation (Bennett & Xie 1988) and partial nerve severing (Seltzer et al 1990). In these studies the degree of pain is inferred from deviation from normal behaviour patterns, e.g. feeding, drinking, grooming and socialising. Clinical models of chronic pain have included arthritis (Vasseur et al 1995) and chronic lameness in sheep and cattle (Ley et al 1995, 1996). In the latter, up-regulation of the central nervous system and hypersensitivity have been demonstrated. The implication is that in animals with long-standing pathology, a defined stimulus creates more neuronal activity than it would in normal animals and this activity lowers the pain threshold and necessitates higher doses of analgesics to control the pain. The foregoing has important implications with regard to the control of chronic pain.

The difficulties discussed earlier (chapter 4) in relation to acute pain are even more relevant when dealing with chronic pain. Subtle abnormalities indicating discomfort may be overlooked without a good knowledge of an animal's normal behaviour. Close questioning of the carer regarding the animal's behaviour patterns, appetite and sleeping patterns should be undertaken. This should particularly concentrate on long-term changes in behaviour. Considerable discomfort may not become apparent until such changes in behaviour have been uncovered and other causes eliminated.

If hypersensitivity occurs, chronic pain will be more difficult to control than acute pain *per se*, requiring either more potent drugs, more frequent doses, longer-acting drugs and/or higher doses. An atypical response to analgesia may indicate that the problem is more long-standing than the carer or veterinarian initially believed. If treatment is palliative rather than curative, long-standing symptomatic analgesia will be required. This raises the ethical problem of the side-effects of chronic dosing with such drugs as opioids (dependency and/or tolerance) and non-steroidal antiinflammatory drugs (gastrointestinal ulceration, renal failure, platelet dysfunction), which are rarely of significance when treating acute pain.

Treatment options

Treatment options are limited in veterinary medicine, partially due to a failure to develop appropriate techniques. Until recently, and still currently in some quarters, the effect of chronic pain on the quality of life in animals has not been recognised, and so treatment has not been required. If it has been recognised then the most popular option has often been euthanasia with the words, 'It is the kindest thing to do' or 'We had better put X out of his/her misery'. However, with increased improvements in cancer therapy in human medicine, and the heightened awareness by the general population of treatment options for chronic conditions, veterinary surgeons will be requested for alternatives to euthanasia. In these circumstances, it is hard, and possibly insensitive, to advise euthanasia for a pet as the kindest option when a relative may be suffering from the same condition. However, as veterinary surgeons we should always remember that our first responsibility is to the animal and not the owner. It is becoming more acceptable and often advisable to apply novel treatments and treatment options originally developed in man to animals but quality of life and relief of suffering must remain our primary concern, rather than merely prolongation of life. Therefore, owners may require very sensitive counselling, particularly if they have projected emotions from personal relationships onto their pet.

There are certain prerequisites for chronic pain relief:

1. The technique or drug administration should not require veterinary knowledge
2. It should be easily applied in the animal's home surroundings by the carer
3. It should not be dangerous for the carer, society or the animal
4. If requiring veterinary skills, the effects should last days and not hours, thus only needing periodic attendance at the veterinary surgery
5. It should be acceptable to carer, veterinary surgeon and the animal.

The present treatment options are outlined below and their applicability to veterinary medicine discussed.

Analgesic agents

Not only is there a wide range of analgesic drugs but also a range of means of administration of the compounds. Not all are used in veterinary medicine at present but they may be in the future.

Routes of administration

1. *Oral dosing* is in some respects the easiest method of drug administration. If the carer can administer medicines orally, then up to three times daily chronic administration is practicable. This is suitable for either sustained release com-

pounds or drugs with longer than 8 hours effective duration. Problems may occur with drugs which have a shorter duration of action than that suggested from their plasma half-life. Thus, the desired action of the drug may only occur above a certain plasma concentration, but the drug will continue to be in the body for some time after the cessation of the desired effect. An example of this would be thiopentone sodium. Recovery of consciousness from this drug mainly occurs by redistribution of thiopentone sodium to body fat, but due to its slow metabolism the drug remains in the body for some time after return of consciousness. Repeat dosing with such a drug may require increasing the periods between doses or giving a loading dose followed by a lower maintenance dose (see Fig. 6.1). Therefore, a knowledge of the particular drug and its pharmacokinetics in that species is required to avoid overdosing or underdosing. A clear example of species differences in this respect is the use of aspirin in dogs and cats. In dogs the recommended dosing interval is 8–12 hours; in cats it is once every 48 hours to achieve a similar plasma concentration of salicylic acid, the active metabolite of aspirin (Potthoff & Carithers 1989).

Problems arise if the dose required is difficult to measure out due to the relatively large size of the tablet in relation to the dose needed or if the animal is difficult to dose orally. However, although there may be a generally available formulation, further examination of formularies will frequently bring to light alternative oral formulations, e.g. paediatric suspension rather than tablets. These may be easier to divide up into doses suitable for small animals, or easier to administer to the animal.

2. Administration by *subcutaneous injection* can be taught to owners quite easily as demonstrated by the successful home treatment of insulin-dependent diabetics.

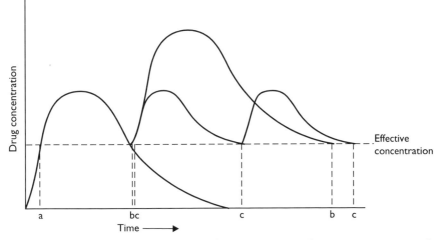

Figure 6.1 Pharmacokinetics of repeat dosing. a–b Time of effective action; increases with equal multiple doses, assuming simple pharmacokinetics. a–c Time of effective action with loading doses and subsequent maintenance doses.

Good technique and a non-irritant formulation is required so that the animal does not develop an aversion to the injections. Ideally the injections should be required only once or twice a day with a relatively small volume and should be easily injected through a very fine needle to minimise discomfort. The injections should be followed by a suitable reward, e.g. a favourite food or extra attention, so that the animal associates the procedure with some pleasurable event.

3. *Intramuscular injections* are less practicable to teach owners of dogs and cats. In man, intramuscular catheters can be chronically implanted to avoid repeated intramuscular injections while still allowing self-administration. These have not been tested in the veterinary clinical setting.

4. *Intravenous injections* are generally reserved for the rapid control of pain, e.g. intraoperative pain breakthrough, and are not really applicable to the control of chronic pain. However, in man chronically implanted devices are occasionally used to allow patient-controlled analgesia or continuous infusions of analgesic according to a calculated dose rate. Again, these have not found veterinary clinical acceptance so far.

5. *Chronic epidural administration* has similar problems as those associated with intravenous administration. Infection is the major problem with this route, and the consequences of this are very serious. Epidurally administered morphine can provide good analgesia for over 12 hours and may be used in a hospital for pain relief for several days but is impractical in the home setting.

6. *Rectal administration* of some non-steroidal antiinflammatory agents is common in people perioperatively. This route avoids direct gastric irritation by the drugs and is easy to administer. In veterinary medicine, however, this has not been properly evaluated.

7. *Transdermal administration* of fentanyl has been relatively widely used in North America (Robinson et al 1999). Fentanyl is available in various dose patches, e.g. Durogesic 25 (Janssen-Cilag) releases approximately 25 µg/hour for 72 hours; 50 µg and 100 µg patches are also available (see chapters 3 and 7). These should be applied to clean shaved skin under an occlusive dressing. The patch should be so positioned to avoid interference by the animal, as accidental oral dosing will result in overdosage; between the shoulder blades is the commonest site for administration. The patches should not be divided as this may result in accidental human exposure. Robinson et al (1999) suggest covering the release membrane with a non-porous material to reduce the surface available for release, in order to reduce the dose. The advantage of these patches is that they can be applied at the veterinary surgery every few days, require little owner maintenance and provide opioid analgesia. The disadvantage is that, in common with many opioid drugs, they are controlled drugs, they are not licensed for veterinary use, and there is a risk of the patch being eaten by accident, either by the animal or the owners' children. There are also concerns over the disposal of the patches and the potential for human abuse, as with all pure opioids.

Therefore, at the moment they cannot be recommended for animals outside the hospital environment.

8. Use of *sustained release preparations*. Slow release preparations of analgesics are available for use in man. For example, morphine is available in a sustained release form both as an injection (Duromorph) and as tablets (MST). There are no equivalent veterinary products available at present. If the use of a medical preparation is contemplated then the effect of the formulation must be noted in its prescription (see chapter 3).

Analgesia for chronic pain therapy

Opioids

Opioids are traditionally thought to be the ultimate in systemic analgesics, but this is not always true. Some animals will be exquisitely sensitive to opioids and others (particularly those which have been in pain for some time) may show a disappointing response to standard analgesic doses. These animals should not be maintained on an analgesic which obviously provides inadequate pain relief. Alternatives should be tried so as to find a regime which suits the individual. This may involve increasing the dose, changing the drug, changing to another class of analgesic, or combining drugs from different classes. For example, some individuals may show little response to methadone, but be very much more relaxed and show fewer signs of pain when given morphine. Other animals may be more comfortable on a non-steroidal antiinflammatory drug than an opioid or respond more positively to combined treatment. The response should be gauged and the treatment guided by the carer, as well as the experience of the prescribing veterinary surgeon.

Once a drug regimen is found which provides relief for the animal, the most convenient means of administration should be established. Thus, an animal may be given morphine every 3–4 hours intramuscularly for cancer pain and remain relatively comfortable with a good appetite and mobility. Whilst this is practical in the short term in a hospital, it may not be acceptable for the animal in the long term due to the discomfort of injections and fear of this procedure. Repeated morphine injection is impractical at home because of the problems of allowing the owner access to a controlled drug and the frequency of intramuscular injections. Oral administration, particularly with food, may be more acceptable to the animal and technically much easier, but the problem of dispensing a controlled drug still remains.

As all the pure opioid agonists are controlled drugs without veterinary licenses, the individual veterinary surgeon must weigh up the risks to the individual, the community and to the veterinary surgeons' right to prescribe, when prescribing such drugs for owner administration.

Of the partial agonists, buprenophine and butorphanol are the must widely used, and both have veterinary product licenses. Nalbuphine and pentazocine are also available, but are only licensed for use in man. Of these, only butor-phanol is *not* a controlled drug. Butorphanol is available in an injectable form for subcutaneous, intramuscular and intravenous administration. The oral form is marketed principally as an antitussive but can be used for analgesia as well at 0.4–1.0 mg/kg orally in dogs. It has been used at doses of 0.2–1.0 mg/kg orally in cats every 4–5 hours for chronic pain relief. A problem when using this analgesic, and other opioids, is that it can produce sedation and temperament changes which may not be acceptable to the owner.

Non-steroidal antiinflammatory drugs

Non-steroidal antiinflammatory drugs (NSAIDs) have been the mainstay of chronic pain relief in veterinary and human medicine for many years. Many horses and older dogs and cats with osteoarthritis would have been killed much earlier in their lives if these drugs had not been available. These drugs are particularly useful in conditions in which inflammation is a major cause of the pain as, in the main, they are cyclooxygenase inhibitors (see chapter 3).

NSAIDs have two major disadvantages: their side-effects and their widespread availability. The latter problem – familiarity – tends to promote the feeling that this class of drugs is mainly effective in mild pain and is not effective in controlling severe pain. Any person suffering from arthritis will repudiate this assumption, as arthritic pain can be extremely debilitating and is often substantially ameliorated by the use of an NSAID. The current vogue for the use of non-steroidal agents for the treatment of postoperative pain in man and animals also points to their effectiveness. Their use in animals with cancer pain is not so well accepted, partially because the acceptability of treatment of cancer is relatively recent, and also because of the common misconception that only opioids should be used in cancer pain – 'It requires a strong analgesic because the pain is severe'. However, in the authors' experience, good control of the clinical signs of pain, improved appetite and mobility have been reported by owners after treatment of their animals with NSAIDs, and with carprofen in particular. This is despite little change in the original disease condition.

The side-effects of the NSAIDs sometimes limit their use. These include gastrointestinal ulceration and bleeding, renal dysfunction and platelet dysfunction. These effects arise from the effect of the traditional NSAIDs on cyclooxygenase-mediated production of prostaglandins (see chapter 3). In man, the risk of developing gastrointestinal side-effects is minimised by administering NSAIDs with food, in enteric-coated formulations and by the concomitant administration of gastrointesinal protectants. The latter drugs range from sucralfate to misoprostol in order of increasing efficacy and cost. Sucralfate (Antepsin, Wyeth) is a mixture of aluminium hydroxide and sucrose sulphate and is indicated in the prevention and treatment of duodenal ulcers but has also been shown to have some effect on the healing of gastric ulcers. At low pH the compound forms a polymer gel which binds to ulcer craters, preventing further damage and allowing healing to progress. It has also been suggested that sucralfate stimulates the formation of prostaglandins by the gastric mucosa, thus resulting in a cytoprotective effect. The recommended dose for dogs is 0.25–1.00 g three times and day and that for cats is 250 mg two to three times daily.

The histamine-2 (H_2) receptor antagonists are very widely used in the treatment of gastrointestinal ulceration. These drugs act by competitively blocking histamine receptors on the gastric parietal cells which secrete acid, and this reduction in acid production allows the ulcer to heal. Of the available compounds ranitidine has the least side-effects and is probably the drug of choice. The dose for dogs is 2 mg/kg twice daily orally or by intravenous injection.

Omeprazole inhibits gastric acid secretion by inhibiting the proton pump. This is a rather more subtle mechanism of action than an H_2 inhibitor, as omeprazole's action is proton pump function-dependent. The dose of this drug is 0.5–1.0 mg/kg orally once daily.

The final type of drug in this armamentarium is the prostaglandin analogue, misoprostol (Cytotec, Searle). The specific indication for this drug is NSAID-induced ulceration. It is a synthetic prostaglandin E_1 analogue and, in effect, replaces the hormone inhibited by NSAIDs in the gut and hence prevents the deleterious effects of its absence. Its high price precludes its routine use, but it should be considered in animals with a history of NSAID intolerance, animals with high circulating corticosteroid concentrations and those prone to gastrointestinal ulceration who may be receiving NSAID therapy. The dose in horses is 0.5 μg/kg four times daily and that in dogs is 2–5 μg/kg three times daily. An excellent description of the use of the gastrointestinal protective drugs in man is provided by Dutta and Sood (1994).

Other drugs which may assist in providing pain relief

Corticosteroid drugs should not be ignored as analgesics. These drugs are extremely effective and it is generally their side-effect of predisposing to hypoadrenocorticism which limits their full use (see chapter 3). However, in chronic or terminal conditions the development of iatrogenic Cushing's disease may well be preferable to suffering from chronic pain.

Mood-altering drugs, e.g. tricyclic antidepressants (TCAD), monoamine oxidase inhibitors (MAOI) and benzodiazepines can all provide relief of chronic pain. In man, it is recognised that there is an increased incidence of clinical depression in patients suffering from chronic pain. In some studies, treatment with MAOI or TCAD drugs relieve both the chronic pain and the clinical depression (Jenkins et al 1976, MacNeill & Dick 1976). However, there is evidence to suggest that they have an analgesic effect separate from their antidepressant effects (e.g. Puttini et al 1986). These effects are mediated via the drugs' action on central catecholamine and indolamine neurotransmitter systems which are also involved in the effects of opioids. However, there are no published reports of the use of these classes of drugs in the treatment of chronic pain in veterinary clinical cases and so their effectiveness in animals must remain speculative. In contrast, the benzodiazepines, with their muscle relaxant properties, are very effective in treating pain in veterinary patients in which muscle spasm contributes to the pain experience, e.g. chronic back pain. However, owners should be warned of the potential behaviour changes and, in some cases, this effect may render the drugs unacceptable to owners, despite causing some amelioration of symptoms.

Local anaesthetic techniques, whilst excellent for acute pain relief, cannot be used easily long-term. Local analgesia is useful to test whether more permanent desensitisation would be of use, e.g. the use of local analgesia of the infraorbital nerve prior to neurectomy as a treatment for head shaking in horses.

Combining drugs with different modes of actions can be extremely successful as there are often synergistic effects, allowing reduced doses of each individual drug to be used for a given effect. This has the added advantage of reducing the side-effects of each individual drug. Of the classes of drugs mentioned, only two should not be combined: the non-steroidal antiinflammatory agents and cortico-steroids, as these drugs act sequentially on the inflammatory cascade, steroids acting on phospholipase and NSAIDs on cyclooxygenase. As these drugs act on the same pathway, their side-effects are at least additive; thus, the risk of gastrointestinal haemorrhage and damage are greatly increased if they are given simultaneously.

Physical techniques for chronic pain therapy

Sensory neurectomy

Sectioning of sensory nerves will abolish all sensation for the supplied area and so may be useful in intractable, incurable pain. For example, for many years the symptomatic treatment of navicular disease in horses has been neurectomy. However, there are several side-effects of such desensitisation, the major being that accidental injury with consequent tissue damage becomes asymptomatic. Therefore, the carer must be extremely vigilant and examine the desensitised area regularly for evidence of damage and/or infection. The second problem is the development of neuromas at the end of the sectioned nerve. These present as painful swellings in the area of the surgery. In themselves they are benign but they cause problems due to the pain which arises from them (neuropathic pain). Neurectomy may be achieved either by surgery or local injection of a toxic chemical such as absolute alcohol or phenol to ablate the nerve.

Therapeutic surgery

This generally involves physical removal of the stimulus causing the pain, e.g. removal of prolapsed intervertebral disc material causing spinal cord or nerve root compression or removal of a tumour which is releasing inflammatory mediators. This is the ultimate in pain control although perioperative analgesics will also be required to ameliorate the acute pain associated with surgery. Removal of the cause is always more satisfactory than mere control of the pain symptoms, but this is not possible in all cases and in rare conditions pain continues despite removal of the inciting cause. A popularly quoted example of this is phantom limb pain after an amputation in man. However, this is often not strictly a sensation of pain which persists after removal of the limb. Sectioning of a peripheral nerve results in a spectrum of sensations ranging from awareness of the denervated part to painful sensations arising from the amputated extremity, including painful sensations from the site of the amputation. Whether this occurs in animals cannot be known with certainty but there is no reason to suppose animals are fundamentally different to man. Some animals, following amputation of a limb, will compulsively lick or otherwise interfere with the site of the amputation long after wound healing is complete, suggesting that they are experiencing a sensation from the site of the amputation. As far as the authors are aware no concerted attempt has been made to treat this phenomenon in animals.

Physiotherapy

Unless the veterinarian has had specific training in physiotherapy, it is preferable to recruit a trained physiotherapist for the application of this method of treatment, as these professionals have a greater understanding of its uses and limitations. For example, laser and ultrasound treatments can exacerbate some conditions if used incorrectly. Ideally, the physiotherapist should be a member of the Association of Chartered Physiotherapists with training in animal treatment. Treatment options available include heat, cold, massage, controlled passive and active exercise, ultrasound and laser therapy. These are generally most effective in orthopaedic disorders in which some aspect of muscle spasm may be involved in the production of pain. For further details interested readers should contact a trained physiotherapist.

Stimulation-induced analgesia

These therapies utilise the patient's endogenous mechanisms for minimising pain either by stimulation of subsets of afferent nerve fibres (non-painful paraesthesia) or by stimulation of release of circulating endorphins (extra-segmental painful stimuli). Stimulation of afferent nerve fibres activates inhibitory mechanisms within the dorsal horn of the spinal cord. Low threshold electrical stimulation or mechanical vibration of peripheral receptors is used to fire the afferent fibres. The stimulation is applied to the area of the body in which the pain is located, unlike acupuncture which is applied extra-segmentally.

The commonest means of applying non-painful paraesthesia is by transcutaneous electrical nerve stimulation (TENS). Other means available are peripheral stimulation by implanted electrodes (subcutaneous or direct contact with the nerve), antidromic activation of afferents by direct stimulation of the dorsal columns of the spinal cord and mechanical stimulation by the application of a vibrator to the skin. TENS is applied by surface electrodes. The electrodes must make good electrical contact with the skin to decrease skin impedance and thus avoid burns. To this end the hair should be clipped and degreased prior to the application of the electrodes. Self-adhesive electrodes are available but are manufactured for man and so adhesion to animal skin can be a problem. Elecrolyte-impregnated gel (e.g. ECG gel) may improve contact. Typical ranges of stimulation characteristics are current 0–50 mA, frequency 0–100 Hz and pulse duration 0.1–0.5 ms. Because chronic pain in animals is so poorly recognised there are few reports of the use of this treatment in animals but hopefully this will change in future and more critical appraisal of its use will become available.

Acupuncture is a well-recognised and widely used means of providing acute pain relief in man and has its advocates for the amelioration of chronic pain but the remarks made with regard to TENS also apply to this pain-relieving modality. Unlike TENS, acupuncture is thought to act via diffuse noxious inhibitions control (DNIC), with the stimulation of certain points of the body causing such an intense response that a type of stress–induced analgesia results. Further details on acupuncture can be found in Schoen (1994) or in the other information sources on acupuncture given at the end of this chapter.

Radiation therapy

Radiation therapy may be administered either with curative intent or as a palliative treatment. The primary aim of definitive radiation therapy is to secure extension of life by long-term control of a tumour or to produce complete remission. In itself, this will provide relief of pain and discomfort as a result of the physical reduction in the size of the tumour. Palliative radiation therapy aims to provide relief of pain and the dysfunction which resulted from the cancer (Richter & Coia 1985), and a secondary benefit is the extension of life. A common use of palliative radiotherapy in man is for the treatment of pain associated with tumour metastases to bone and it has been used in a similar manner in dogs to control pain associated with bone tumours. Osteosarcoma of the long bones in dogs is a most painful condition which is often refractory to analgesic drug therapy. Amputation (followed by adjuvant chemotherapy) is the definitive treatment and is well tolerated by giant and heavy breeds such as Wolfhounds and Rottweilers. However, radiation can be used as a palliative therapy when the owner is reluctant to accept the option of amputation or if there are medical contraindications to this treatment (e.g. 'wobbler' syndrome). Radiation therapy can achieve pain relief in about two-thirds of dogs, with a median survival of about 5 months (c.f. 10 months for amputation plus adjuvant chemotherapy). Pathological fracture at the tumour site is a potential complication of this treatment if the dog starts weight bearing (this is especially true for the more lytic tumours) and this may then necessitate amputation or euthanasia. The mechanism whereby radiation achieves pain relief is poorly understood but it can occur following only one dose of radiation.

Euthanasia

There are times when, despite the best intentions and best efforts of the veterinarian, the pain and suffering of an individual animal cannot be relieved.

Euthanasia then becomes the only humane option. In other circumstances, euthanasia may be offered as an alternative to palliative therapy. Whenever euthanasia is advised it should be done so in a positive manner – 'Euthanasia is a great kindness and Suzie will be at peace'. Compare this with the defeatist and negative attitude of 'There is nothing left to do, so we had better put her to sleep'. This will be the final decision the owner will have to make for their living pet companion and so should be handled sympathetically. Following the death of a pet, owners move through the various stages of bereavement – grief, anger and blame. The circumstances under which euthanasia is advised, and performed, can heighten or diminish these emotions. Euthanasia is a privilege that we as veterinarians can exercise but it should not be undertaken lightly. To advise and perform euthanasia without explaining other options or the reasons can have serious consequences. An owner who later discovered that there was another option may become aggressive and litigious, even although the alternative was not really sensible. There are many papers written about euthanasia in veterinary practice but the article by Guntzelman and Riegger (1993) presents a good overview with much practical advice.

References

Bennett, G.J. and Xie, Y. (1988) A peripheral mono-neuropathy in rat that produces disorders of pain sensation like those seen in man. *Pain* **33**: 87–107.

Colpaert, F.C. (1987) Evidence that adjuvant arthritis in the rat is associated with chronic pain. *Pain* **28**: 201–222.

Craig, K.D. (1994) Emotional aspects of pain. In: Wall, P.D. and Melzack, R. (eds) *Textbook of Pain*. Churchill Livingstone, Edinburgh, ch 13, pp 261–274.

De Castro Costa, M., De Sutter, P., Gybels, J. and Van Hees, J. (1981) Adjunct-induced arthritis in rats: a possible animal model of chronic pain. *Pain* **10**: 173–185.

Dutta, S.K. and Sood, R. (1994) Clinical pharmacology of drugs used in GI disorders of critically ill patients. In: Chernow, B. (ed) *The Pharmacological Approach to the Critically Ill Patient*. Williams and Wilkins, Baltimore.

Guntzelman, J. and Riegger, M.H. (1993) Helping pet owners with the euthanasia decision. *Veterinary Medicine* **88**: 26–34.

Iadarola, M.J., Brady, L.S., Draisci, G. and Dubner R. (1988) Enhancement of dynophin gene expression in spinal cord following experimental inflammation stimulus. Specificity, behavioural parameters and opioid receptor binding. *Pain* **32**: 77–88.

Jenkins, D.G., Ebbutt, A.F. and Evans, C.D. (1976) Imipramine in treatment of low back pain. *Journal of International Medical Research* 4(**2**): 28–40.

Ley, S.J., Waterman, A.E. and Livingston, A. (1995) A field study of the effect of lameness on mechanical nociceptive thresholds in sheep. *Veterinary Record* 137(**4**): 85–87.

Ley, S.J., Waterman, A.E. and Livingston, A. (1996) Measurement of mechanical thresholds, plasma cortisol and catecholamines in control and lame cattle: a preliminary study. *Research in Veterinary Science* 61(**2**): 172–173.

MacNeill, A.L. and Dick, W.C. (1976) Imipramine and rheumatoid factor. *Journal of Internal Medicine Research* 4(**2**): 23–27.

Potthoff, A. and Carithers, R.W. (1989) Pain and analgesia in dogs and cats. *Compendium for Continuing Education in Veterinary Medicine: Small Animals* 11(**8**): 887–897.

Puttini, P.S., Cazzola, M., Boccasini, L. et al (1986) A comparison of dothiepin versus placebo in the treatment of pain in rheumatoid arthritis and the association of pain with depression. *Journal of International Medical Research* **16**: 331–337.

Ren, K. and Dubner, R. (1999) Inflammatory models of pain and hyperalgesia. *International Laboratory Animal Research Journal*, **40**: 111–118.

Richter, M.P. and Coia, L.R. (1985) Palliative radiation therapy. *Seminars in Oncology* **12**: 375–383.

Robinson, T.M., Kruse-Elliott, K.T., Markel, M.D. et al (1999) A comparison of transdermal fentanyl versus epidural morphine for analgesia in dogs undergoing major orthopaedic surgery. *Journal of the American Animal Hospital Association* **35**: 95–100.

Schoen, A.M. (ed) (1994) *Veterinary Acupuncture: Ancient Art to Modern Medicine*. Mosby, St. Louis.

Seltzer, Z., Dubner, R. and Shir, Y. (1990) A novel behavioural model of neuropathic pain disorders produced in rats by partial sciatic nerve injury. *Pain* **43**: 205–218.

Sternbach, R.A. (1981) Chronic pain as a disease entity. *Triangle* 20(**1/2**): 27–32.

Vasseur, P.B., Johnson, A.L. Budsberg, S.C. et al (1995) Randomized, controlled trial of the efficacy of carprofen, a non-steroidal anti-inflammatory drug in the treatment of osteoarthritis in dogs. *Journal of the American Veterinary Medicine Association* 206(**6**): 807–812.

Weisenberg, M. (1994) Cognitive aspects of pain. In: Wall, P.D. and Melzack, R. (eds) *Textbook of Pain*. Churchill Livingstone, Edinburgh, ch 14, pp 275–289.

Information sources on acupuncture

- *Complimentary and Alternative Veterinary Medicine: Principles and Practice.* edited by Allen M. Schoen and Susan G. Wynn (Mosby, St. Louis, 1998).
- pva-1 (professional veterinary acupuncture list). To subscribe, send email to: listserv@med.auth.gr with the command 'subscribe' in the main body text. No subject, no signature. Archives are at: http: //users.med.auth.gr/localsrv/lists/pa-1/
- IVAS (International Veterinary Acupuncture Society), IVAS Office PO Box 178, Longmont, CO 80502–1478. email: ivasoffice@aol.com
- Association of British Veterinary Acupuncture – address varies, contact RCVS.
- Acupuncture Progress [titles and abstracts] at: http://users.med.auth.gr/~karanik/english/acuprog.html
- Acubase – CNUSC, France [titles only; *no* abstracts] at: http://www.cnusc.fr/
- Acupuncture References [A bibliography of 2302 *titles* (not abstracts), Jan 1970 to Oct 1997, by L.J. Klein & A.I. Trachtenberg, USDH/NIH/NLM/NIDA] at: http://www.nlm.nih.gov/pubs/cbm/acupuncture.html

PROBLEMS OF PAIN MANAGEMENT

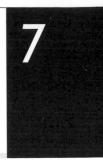

P.J. Pascoe

Pain management scenarios

Patient presented following trauma

Animals presented to the veterinarian immediately after a traumatic event may or may not be in pain. This somewhat contradictory statement is based on data from man where it has been shown that a significant proportion of patients have a pain-free period immediately following trauma (Melzack et al 1982). However, there are also a significant number of patients that are in pain immediately after the injury and it is very difficult, when dealing with animals that cannot directly report their pain, to determine which is the case. With this in mind it is generally advisable to give an analgesic as soon as the animal has been examined. In some cases the addition of an analgesic may facilitate the examination since the animal may guard the area fiercely because of the pain. The best drugs to use, in this circumstance, are the opioids since they have a short onset time and provide potent analgesia. Many of the opioids can be given intravenously so they can be titrated to effect in these patients. In some species (e.g. dog), rapid intravenous injection of morphine or pethidine (meperidine) should be avoided because of the risk of hypotension (see chapter 3). Although this may be tolerated in a healthy patient, trauma cases, particularly those with cardiovascular instability, may be at greater risk.

In patients in hypovolaemic shock it is best to treat the shock at the same time. If the animal appears to be in pain during the resuscitation, the opioid should be administered carefully because the drug may have much more profound effects than in the normal patient due to altered drug pharmacokinetics. The rate of i.v. administration should be tailored to the particular drug being used and the response of the animal. For example, alfentanil reaches its peak effect within 1-2 minutes whereas oxymorphone may take up to 8 minutes to reach its maximum effect. The administration of μ opioids in patients with concomitant septic/endotoxic shock may be contraindicated since there is extensive experimental evidence to suggest that the opioid antagonist, naloxone, may improve cardiac output, blood pressure and utilisation of lactate during septic/endotoxic shock (Hinshaw et al 1984). This has also been shown to be true with moderate doses of nalbuphine (an opioid agonist-antagonist). In one canine haemorrhagic shock study, nalbuphine, at doses of 1–4 mg/kg plus 1–4 mg/kg/hour improved haemodynamics and survival while higher doses (8 mg/kg and 8 mg/kg/h) had negative effects on both parameters (Hunt et al 1984).

Once initial treatment of the patient has been completed, a decision needs to be made as to how the pain will be controlled over the next 24–48 hours. In cases with relatively minor trauma it may be unnecessary to use further analgesia. In moderate trauma a regime of intermittent administration of opioids may be sufficient, with the dosing interval tailored for the drug and the response of the patient. The variation in requirement for analgesics is a multilayered issue since it will be influenced by the genetics of the animal, its previous experiences, the current environment and the degree of trauma it has suffered. In human patients analgesia is often provided by a technique known as 'patient controlled analgesia' (PCA). With this method patients are able to control their pain by pressing a button which is connected to a pump containing an analgesic. When the button is pressed a predetermined dose of drug is given and then the pump will usually prevent further administration of the drug for a period which corresponds to the peak onset of the analgesic, thus preventing patients from overdosing themselves. Looking at the range of doses self-administered by patients following similar procedures provides a powerful illustration of the variation in individual analgesic requirements. In one relatively small study (15 patients) the amount of morphine given over the first 24 hours after a craniotomy ranged from 2 to 79 mg (Stoneham et al 1996)!

Patients with severe trauma may need a continuous regime and an opioid infusion may be useful in providing background analgesia, always with the proviso that more can be given if the animal appears to be painful. Some cases like this may benefit from a fentanyl patch since this provides a relatively constant plasma concentration of the drug. The patch should be applied as soon as possible and systemic opioids given for about 24 hours in dogs and 12 hours in cats, since this is the time it takes for plasma concentrations of fentanyl to rise to a 'steady state' (see chapter 3). Even though the patch has been applied and sufficient time allowed for plasma concentrations to reach 'steady state', the animal may still need supplemental analgesic therapy and should be treated if signs of pain are present. NSAIDs may be used for long-term pain control in these patients as long as there are only relatively minor changes in circulatory function. These drugs should be avoided in patients with hypovolaemia or unstable haemodynamics because their effects on gastric and renal circulation are likely to be exacerbated, resulting in gastric ulceration and/or renal insufficiency. If the patient is going to undergo surgery, an NSAID should be chosen that is not likely to interfere with platelet function. Most of these drugs affect platelet production of thromboxane A_2 which is essential for platelet aggregation and the formation of a stable clot (Schafer 1995). Aspirin acetylates this site and so causes a permanent change while other NSAIDs affect this site only while the drug is active in the circulation. Consequently a dose of aspirin will affect platelet activity for 5–8 days (it takes this period of time for new platelets to be made) while long-acting NSAIDs may affect platelet aggregation for 2–3 days (e.g. piroxicam, naproxen, diclofenac and indomethacin); the effects from drugs with short half-lives (e.g.

ibuprofen) may only last 24 hours (Schafer 1995). If surgery is expected to take place in less than a week then aspirin should be avoided. If surgery is expected to take place within 24–72 hours an NSAID with an appropriate half-life should be chosen. Carprofen may be an exception in that it has very weak activity in inhibiting thromboxane A_2 (McKellar et al 1990, Taylor et al 1996). In canine studies no inhibition was evident at doses up to 4 mg/kg while in cats a low dose caused no change but there was mild inhibition at 4 mg/kg. Some trauma victims may be especially prone to the effects of NSAID on platelets because of blood loss and/or coagulopathies associated with the trauma and shock.

Raised intracranial pressure

The main issue in this situation is that intracranial pressure (ICP) is dependent on the volume of brain tissue, the volume of the CSF and the volume of the blood within the cranium. Routine therapies using mannitol or furosemide (frusemide) are aimed at reducing the volume of tissue and CSF in the cranial vault but short-term control of intracranial pressure is dependent on the volume of blood within the cranium. Cerebral blood flow is directly related to $PaCO_2$; anything which depresses ventilation is likely to increase $PaCO_2$ with a resultant increase in cerebral blood flow and therefore ICP. Pain itself may tend to increase intracranial pressure and the effective control of pain may help to reduce ICP. Opioids in relatively low doses do not seem to cause significant respiratory depression in normal dogs and cats but the effects may be exacerbated in an animal with depressed mentation due to an increased ICP. The clinician should therefore be very careful with the use of these drugs in this situation. In our clinic opioids are commonly used for premedication of patients with a suspected increase in ICP with normal to slightly depressed mentation but are avoided in those animals that are obtunded or comatose. In the setting where the animal needs to be given analgesics for many hours it may be better to use an NSAID. In head trauma cases where the use of an NSAID may be a concern due either to circulatory instability or alterations in blood clotting the clinician should look for local methods of pain control. If the animal has pain in its hind quarters an epidural with morphine and/or bupivacaine may provide relief. Morphine at the doses used for epidural analgesia is very unlikely to cause respiratory depression and even if it does it is possible to reverse the systemic depression with naloxone while maintaining the local analgesia. An epidural injection with morphine may be helpful for chest or front limb trauma but the effects are likely to be less predictable than for the hind limb. Local anaesthetic blocks should also be considered for any area that would be accessible for such techniques.

Severe unremitting pain following surgery

Animals with severe pain following surgery should be evaluated for signs of nerve entrapment. If a nerve has been ligated, partially ligated or trapped

beneath an implant it can lead to allodynia or causalgia. This syndrome is characterised by the animal showing signs of pain even when the area is touched
lightly. The definitive treatment for this is to reoperate to free the entrapped
nerve but in the meantime the animal should be treated with a continuous infusion of an opioid with the addition of an NSAID (see also treatments for neuropathic pain). In animals that have undergone extremely invasive or prolonged
surgery the use of opioid infusions is also warranted. The author typically uses
morphine but other opioids are likely to be just as effective. A loading dose of
0.5 mg/kg is drawn up and this is diluted to 20–30 ml with saline and then given
over 5–10 minutes. This is done to avoid the histamine release commonly associated with rapid i.v. injection of morphine. An infusion is then started at 0.1–1.0
mg/kg/h. In most cases the author starts at 0.2 mg/kg/h and then increases or
decreases the infusion rate according to the signs displayed by the animal. For
other opioids the dose normally used for a given period can be divided up and
given as an infusion. For example, if methadone was the drug of choice and the
usual dose was 0.4 mg/kg/4 h then the infusion would start at 0.1 mg/kg/h. This
can then be adjusted according to the needs of the patient. In cats, infusions of μ
agonists are likely to be accompanied by excitation and so agonist/antagonists
such as butorphanol can be used. A loading dose of 0.1 mg/kg can be given
intravenously followed by an infusion of 0.03–0.40 mg/kg/h.

A further refinement of this for pain in the front or hind legs or over the
trunk would be to give the drugs by epidural injection. In this instance an
epidural catheter should be placed and the tip of the catheter located close
to the painful dermatome(s). For hind-quarter pain the catheter would be
advanced 1–2 cm beyond the tip of the needle whereas it would be advanced up
into the thoracic region for fore-quarter pain. Once in place the drugs can be
delivered by intermittent injection or by continuous infusion (see chapter 5)

Neuropathic pain

Neuropathic pain involves injury to neuronal tissue which results in sensory
deficits with abnormal pain sensations from the area supplied by the nerve(s) or
from areas influenced by the sensory input (referred pain). In man, neuropathic
pain syndromes are described associated with lesions in the central nervous system. Lesions in the spinothalamic tract of the spinal cord appear to be responsible for many of these cases but brainstem, thalamic and cortical lesions have all
been described which result in neuropathic pain. The pathophysiology of neuropathic pain is still being elucidated (Yaksh & Chaplan 1997). There are some
changes induced by the initial barrage of stimuli associated with the nerve
injury and then the chronic post-nerve injury activity further defines the type
of neuropathic pain that may be perceived by the patient. This may entail neuroma formation and the expression of novel ion channels or receptors within
the affected nerve. There may be involvement of the sympathetic nervous
system, both at these neuromas and at the level of the dorsal root ganglia.

Centrally in the spinal dorsal horn there is a loss of GABAergic and glycinergic neurones and there may be afferent sprouting from the large myelinated afferents from their normal area of termination in lamina III up to lamina I. This latter change may explain some of the hyperaesthesia to touch and also the lack of response of some neuropathic pain to opioid treatment, since there are no opioid receptors on the Aβ fibres. The signs of neuropathic pain in man include such descriptions as: spontaneous, continuous, shooting, paroxysmal, allodynia and hyperalgesia, hyperpathia, referred pain with abnormal pain radiation, abnormal pain duration and wind-up like aftersensations. These signs may be difficult to detect in animals but it is thought that the phenomenon of auto-nomy (self-mutilation) may be one sign of neuropathic pain. Animal models of neuropathic pain involve the surgical ligation of a nerve, the injection of chem-icals which cause nerve injury or the induction of diabetes which induces diabetic neuropathies (Jensen 1996). Animals treated in these ways often have hyperalgesia to both thermal and mechanical stimuli.

The management of neuropathic pain is difficult and there is certainly con-cern that opioids may not be effective. In some animal models there is a sensi-tivity to opioid treatment while the majority respond better to the use of NMDA antagonists and alpha-2 agonists. A recent review article of the use of opioids in people with neuropathic pain suggests that opioids may be effective if they are titrated to a dose providing maximum benefit with acceptable side-effects (Dellemijn 1999). This may be feasible in dogs but it is likely that the side-effects of the opioids in cats would be problematic before a therapeutic dose is achieved. Ketamine (1–2 mg/kg every 4–8 hours) appears to be beneficial in cases where opioids have not been effective and the combination of ketamine and an opioid may provide the most effective therapy (Lauretti et al 1999). Ketamine has also been made up in a paste and applied directly to the affected site. Epidural ketamine at 25 μg/kg/h (continued for 10 days) was effective in a human patient with neuropathic pain associated with sciatic nerve injury (Takahashi et al 1998).

Recently, gabapentin has been shown to be effective in some forms of neuro-pathic pain. This drug is thought to work at voltage-dependent calcium chan-nels, although its mechanism of action is not entirely understood. In an experiment in rats, gabapentin was effective at obtunding dynamic allodynia in a diabetic neuropathy while morphine was ineffective (Field et al 1999). In a number of trials in man, gabapentin has been shown to provide more effective therapy in many neuropathic pain patients than opioids alone (Merren 1998, Rowbotham et al 1998). This drug comes in 100, 300 and 400 mg capsules and as 600 and 800 mg tablets. Doses of 5–35 mg/kg/day have been described with the usual recommendation to split that dose into 2–3 administrations. In the case of small patients the capsules can be opened and the powder given with food. The drug is excreted unchanged in the urine so impaired renal function significantly affects the duration of action of the drug.

Another treatment used in human patients is topical capsaicin. This can pro-duce intense burning sensations when applied in the concentrations used for this therapy and local anaesthetics may be applied to blunt this sensation (Robbins et al 1998). This treatment is used because it is supposed to deplete the neurones of substance P.

A subset of neuropathic pain patients may suffer from what has recently been defined as complex regional pain syndrome (Campbell 1996). This complex syndrome is characterised by involvement of the sympathetic – nervous system such that removal of local or systemic sympathetic activation significantly reduces the perceived pain. These patients often appear to have increased sensitivity to cooling stimuli over the affected area. Diagnosis of complex regional pain syndromes involves removal of the sympathetic activity in the affected area. This can be achieved by block of the relevant sympathetic ganglia with local anaesthetics or by giving an alpha–1 antagonist intravenously. For this purpose phentolamine is given intravenously as a continuous infusion and the patient's response to nociceptive stimuli monitored. Once a diagnosis has been made, treatment involves a surgical or chemical ablation of the relevant sympathetic ganglia or ongoing therapy with oral alpha–1 antagonists (Campbell 1996). There is still controversy about the medical management of human patients with these syndromes and the long-term success rate for therapy has not been good.

Burn pain

Animals that have been burned will have pain associated with the area of burn. In true full-thickness burns the nociceptors are destroyed so there is a loss of sensation in that area, but there is still pain associated with the peripheral areas of such burns where the damage has not been as severe. In these patients it is important to control pain from early in the injury period because the continuous nociceptive input can lead to allodynia and hyperpathia over the burned area. Opioids are generally used as the mainstay of such therapy (van den Broek 1991). The degree of pain will depend on the nature and amount of the burn so the therapy can be tailored accordingly (Kowalske & Tanelian 1997). For relatively minor burns it may be unnecessary to institute any ongoing analgesic therapy, whereas for partial-thickness burns over large areas of the body, the animal is likely to need some continuous form of therapy such as a fentanyl patch or an intravenous infusion of opioid. A recent case report of two burned dogs recommended the use of oral ketamine to provide analgesia. These patients had initially been treated with opioids but had progressive signs of pain which responded to oral ketamine given at 8–12 mg/kg every 6 hours. The dogs did not show any side-effects from these doses of ketamine (Joubert 1998).

Burn patients often need frequent dressing changes and it is important to maximise analgesia during this time to decrease the patient's suffering. In many instances it may be advantageous to use a short-acting anaesthetic regime for these procedures. In man, ketamine has commonly been used for dressing changes and the combination of diazepam and ketamine or zolazepam/ tiletamine (Telazol) may be very useful for dogs and cats. These combinations can be titrated to effect such that the animal may not have to be completely anaesthetised to tolerate the dressing change. It is especially important to titrate drugs to effect in these patients because they may have exaggerated effects with drugs which are highly protein-bound (because of protein loss through the burn surface), or they may be resistant to their action due to repeated administration or changes in the volume of distribution.

NSAIDs are not recommended in the early analgesic management of these patients due to the changes in platelet function which could enhance bleeding and the increased likelihood of gastric/duodenal ulceration associated with the stress of injury. These drugs may be very useful for the later management of pain associated with healing and physiotherapy to attain maximum mobility of the joints and skin (van den Broek 1991).

Regional techniques of analgesia have a limited role in these patients because of the increased risk of infection associated with burn injuries.

Equine colic pain

Visceral pain is different from somatic pain in that it can be induced by stimuli which do not signal tissue damage. Distension of a hollow visceral organ or distension of the capsule of a solid visceral organ can be painful without a resulting tissue pathology. Even without distension, spasm of the intestinal wall (increased wall tension) can cause abdominal discomfort. Activity of visceral nociceptors is considerably enhanced by the release of inflammatory cytokines and some afferents which seem to be silent with normal stimuli become active following inflammation (Cervero 1999). Horses have a gastrointestinal tract which is predisposed to disturbances of a functional or physical nature and abdominal pain (colic) is a frequent reason for requests for veterinary intervention. The management of colic pain is a therapeutic challenge because most of the available drugs interfere with important aspects of the pathophysiology of the disease and may increase mortality if used without due care.

The NSAIDs are frequently used as a first line of treatment of animals which appear to have a spasmodic colic. Drugs such as flunixin and Buscopan Compositum (dipyrone and hyoscine) are widely used for this purpose and often appear to alleviate signs within minutes of their administration (Boatwright et al 1996, Hay & Moore 1997). This miraculous cure may be related to central actions of the NSAID or to changes in intestinal motility which relieve the initiating cause of the pain. The negative side of therapy with these drugs is that they often have long-lasting effects and may mask the progression of the disease. This is particularly the case where there is an inflammatory or endotoxaemic component to the condition. By decreasing the inflammatory enhancement of abdominal signs or antagonising the effects of the endotoxin (flunixin especially), an ischaemic segment of bowel may die completely and even rupture with few signs of pain or circulatory disturbance. This suggests that these drugs should be used at relatively low doses (to shorten their duration of action) and that the animal must be assessed completely each time it is decided to repeat the dose. These drugs do not produce any significant sedation and may not be very effective in the animal that is in great pain when the clinician needs to calm in order to carry out a physical examination (Jochle et al 1989).

The alpha-2 agonists have been used extensively for the management of equine colic and are generally the first drugs of choice in the animal which is uncontrollable and is at the point of hurting itself or injuring its handlers. In severe cases, detomidine is usually the drug of choice because of its potent sedative and analgesic effects (Jochle 1989, Jochle et al 1989, Martin et al 1995). These beneficial effects of the alpha-2 agonists come at the price of some significant effects on other systems in the body. These drugs slow large intestinal motility and while this may be of benefit in a spasmodic colic it may promote dysfunction in an animal with an impaction or may enhance postoperative intestinal ileus (Kohn 1999). They also cause a significant decrease in cardiac output and a peripheral vasoconstriction. These changes in circulatory function may exacerbate problems with circulatory shock and may also increase the risk of ischaemic damage to bowel with restricted circulation (e.g. epiploic foramen entrapment). The alpha-2 agonists can also be profound diuretics and this could contribute further to the circulatory disturbances; however, it is not known whether this effect continues in the face of dehydration. These pharmacological disturbances need to be considered by the clinician managing a horse with colic but should not be a reason to withhold analgesia in the situation where relief could be obtained with these highly potent drugs. Another advantage with these drugs is that their effects can largely be reversed by their antagonists (tolazoline, atipamezole and yohimbine) if it is thought that the effect of the agonist has been detrimental or if the clinician needs to be able to assess the animal in the absence of analgesia.

The opioids are generally not very effective analgesics in horses when used alone but may be useful adjuncts to other therapies. The μ agonists (morphine, methadone, pethidine/meperidine, oxymorphone and the fentanyl derivatives) can cause significant disturbances of intestinal motility and locomotor activity and need to be used cautiously in equine colic (Roger et al 1994). At low doses they may provide additional pain relief when combined with NSAIDs or alpha-2 agonists and in combination with the latter they may make it easier to examine a fractious painful animal (Hay & Moore 1997). The κ agonists (e.g. butorphanol, pentazocine) are less likely to cause disturbances of intestinal motility and locomotor activity and may be better choices in the management of equine colic. Butorphanol can provide adequate analgesia but may be accompanied by some restlessness and shivering at higher doses (0.22 mg/kg) (Kalpravidh et al 1984, Boatwright et al 1996). At 0.1 mg/kg, butorphanol did not appear to be very effective in clinical cases of colic – none of the 10 horses receiving butorphanol had satisfactory pain relief (Jochle et al 1989). Pentazocine did not provide adequate analgesia in a caecal balloon model of visceral pain but may provide some relief in a clinical setting (Lowe 1978). These κ agonists are also best combined with alpha-2 agonists to provide the most effective analgesia and these combinations may also make it easier to examine the horse since they tend to stand better than when either drug is given alone.

Animals which cannot be controlled with the above regimens may need to be sedated in addition to receiving analgesics. Great care and attention needs to be paid if this step is necessary because of the risks of exacerbating shock and hypotension. The horse should be given the least amount of drug to achieve the desired goals. Drugs that could be used would include chloral hydrate, guaifenesin and perhaps even low doses of ketamine (0.1–25.0 mg/kg).

Pancreatic pain

Pancreatitis is a relatively common condition in small animals and is often associated with marked abdominal pain. Opioids are commonly used for the management of this pain but are often not very effective. In man, the opioids are a concern because the bile duct and the main pancreatic duct join together and the fluid is released into the intestine through the sphincter of Oddi. This sphincter tends to constrict with the administration of morphine. Other drugs also cause an increase in sphincter pressure (e.g. methadone, pethidine/meperidine, fentanyl, hydromorphone, pentazocine and butorphanol), but nalbuphine and buprenorphine have minimal effect (Juvara & Radulesco 1967, McCammon et al 1984, Rothuizen et al 1990, Isenhower & Mueller 1998). In dogs, the bile duct and pancreatic duct are usually separate so these concerns are not valid but the two ducts are common in about 80% of cats so it would be best to use nalbuphine or buprenorphine, with butorphanol as the next choice since these analgesics have the least effects on the ducts. In those cases where the opioids do not seem to be effective an epidural technique may be helpful. An epidural catheter should be placed so that the end of the catheter is around T13-L2 and an infusion of bupivacaine, at a dose low enough to cause minimal effect on motor function, plus morphine, may be very effective. Epidural morphine does not appear to affect the pressure in the sphincter of Oddi (Vatashsky et al 1984). NSAIDs may also be of use since part of the pain in these cases is related to an inflammatory component – phospholipase A_2 – being particularly important. However, they have not proven to be very effective except in mild cases (Irving 1997) and many clinicians are concerned about their use in these circumstances because of the possible increased risk for gastric or duodenal ulceration.

Some clinicians have used ketamine for pancreatic pain and have found it to be fairly effective. Doses used have been in the 1–2 mg/kg range (s.c. or i.m. every 4–8 hours).

Excitement during recovery from anaesthesia

Dog

It is not uncommon for dogs recovering from surgery to go through a period of excitement or delirium. This is often a short-lived phenomenon and may just require some physical restraint and soothing for the animal to calm down. However, one contributing factor to this excitement may be pain and it is sometimes difficult to determine whether or not this is the case. When dealing with this situation the first thing to determine is whether the animal is *likely* to be in pain, i.e. has it had an invasive procedure and if so has it received analgesics? If the dog has received an analgesic, was the drug given at such a time that it would have reached its peak effect? For example, if buprenorphine is given immediately before discontinuing an inhalant it is unlikely to be beneficial since it takes at least 30 minutes to be effective (Waterman & Kalthum 1992). If the drug has not had time to reach its peak effect or has not been given then a further dose of opioid should be administered at this stage, intravenously. While NSAIDs may be effective for some early postoperative pain they do not seem to be as effective as opioids and in general have a much longer latency (Lascelles et al 1995).

If the dog continues to be excited and has received what is thought to be adequate analgesic therapy then it is appropriate to use a tranquilliser. This should be given intravenously in low doses (e.g. acepromazine at 0.01 mg/kg). More can be given if necessary but usually this is sufficient to calm the animal. Once the animal is calm it is advisable to assess the surgical site if possible and see if the animal is still very sensitive to manipulation – this may suggest that further analgesic therapy is still warranted. Some animals still do not calm down with this approach and it may be that they are getting agitated from the effects of the opioid. There are two ways of approaching this: give a further dose of short-acting opioid or administer an opioid antagonist. The following protocol is recommended. If there is concern that the animal's behaviour is still motivated by pain, the short-acting opioid (e.g. alfentanil or fentanyl) is given intravenously and the animal watched carefully. If the behaviour dissipates, then the animal can be treated with a longer-acting analgesic but if the behaviour remains or intensifies then it is necessary to give an opioid antagonist. Ideally, a mixed agonist/antagonist is used for this purpose since it will reverse the effect of the μ agonist while leaving the animal with some analgesia from the action at κ receptors. Nalbuphine (0.03–0.10 mg/kg) is an excellent choice for this purpose since it provides adequate reversal, good analgesia and minimal sedation. If a pure antagonist is used it should be one of the shorter-acting drugs such as naloxone. It should be given slowly and titrated until the animal calms down. A dose of 1–10 μg/kg is a good starting point with naloxone. In man, administration of naloxone has been associated with pulmonary oedema but this has usually been the result of giving a high dose rapidly. This problem has not been reported in dogs.

Cat

Although many of the same comments apply to cats, opioid excitation is more predictable in this species if high doses of opioids are used. Nevertheless, there are individual cats that become excited with relatively low doses and these need to be handled in the manner described above. In some cats, particularly after a very invasive procedure, opioid analgesics do not seem to provide sufficient pain relief and the cat will throw itself around the cage in a very self-destructive fashion. These cats do not respond well to acepromazine and the only two methods that have worked for this author are to use either pentobarbital or medetomidine. The latter is my preference in cats that have normal or nearly normal cardiovascular function. Medetomidine is an analgesic and provides profound sedation – a dose of 2–5 µg/kg i.v. is often enough to sedate the animal for long enough for them to recover smoothly. Higher doses or repeated doses are needed in some cases. One big advantage with medetomidine is that if the animal becomes too sedated, or some other problem is noticed, the effect of the drug can be antagonised with atipamezole. Pentobarbital will give profound sedation at doses from 2–10 mg/kg i.v. and again recovery following this treatment is usually much smoother. Pentobarbital is not reversible and the animal will require physiological support if the dose given causes excessive sedation.

Horse

The period of recovery from anaesthesia in the horse is notorious for its potential hazards of excitement and ataxia. It is particularly difficult to differentiate excitement from pain in this period. However, there is no doubt that pain contributes significantly to excitement and distress after anaesthesia (Taylor & Clarke 1999). It is difficult to treat a horse that is thrashing and staggering during recovery, so it is essential to prevent pain as far as possible. Analgesics should be given before anaesthetic delivery is discontinued whenever any surgical or other invasive procedure is undertaken. Opioids may themselves cause agitation, but a single dose of an opioid given before consciousness returns is unlikely to cause a problem. Butorphanol (up to 0.1 mg/kg), particularly if given intramuscularly during surgery, will contribute to postoperative analgesia. A combination of an NSAID and an opioid is probably the best approach. Morphine or other pure µ agonist is more likely to cause excitement than the partial or mixed agonists. Good stabilisation and support of the surgical site will also contribute to analgesia. Local anaesthesia may be used to provide postoperative analgesia in horses, but blocks above the fetlock affect proprioception and will increase incoordination, ataxia and distress whenever the horse stands; hence this approach has limited value for postoperative analgesia in this species.

A full bladder will cause considerable agitation and early attempts to rise. Catheterisation to empty the bladder when the horse is placed in the recovery box will calm the recovery period as much as any analgesic and should always be included after surgery lasting more than 30–60 minutes. Hypoxaemia will also cause restlessness during recovery. A clear airway must be assured and supplementary oxygen given if necessary. Inevitably, in spite of attention to all of the above, a smooth pain-free recovery cannot be guaranteed. It is fairly common practice to sedate horses recovering from volatile agent anaesthesia with alpha-2 adrenoceptor agonists to smooth the return of consciousness. Xylazine (50–100 mg i.v. total dose) is the most commonly used agent. Its main effect is sedative but it may produce its overall effect by enhancing analgesia as well.

Sensitivity to opioids

Some dogs appear to become excited after administration of opioids and so these drugs cannot be used in their usual fashion for pain control. In most cases this sensitivity appears to be to μ opioid agonists, but some animals are sensitive to both μ and κ agonists. For these patients it is appropriate to use more localised techniques or to use NSAIDs. Local techniques would include the use of epidural morphine because the dose of morphine appears to be so low and the rate of absorption so slow that it does not elicit an excitatory response. The use of local anaesthetic techniques would also be effective for these cases. Ideally, a local anaesthetic/analgesic technique should be combined with an NSAID so that one can gain intense analgesia in the immediate postoperative period while providing longer-lasting analgesia with the NSAID.

Ceiling effects with agonist/antagonists

For mild to moderate pain there appear to be few differences between the agonist/antagonist drugs and the pure agonists. However in more severe pain states it is apparent that substantially increasing the dose and/or frequency of administration of an agonist/antagonist may diminish the effect of the drug. It is not fully understood why this happens but it is possible that the antagonist component of the drug is reversing some of the activity of the agonist. If it is difficult to control pain with one of these drugs after giving a high dose it may be best to allow the drug to wear off and change over to an agonist. In the interim an NSAID could be given or a local anaesthetic/analgesic technique applied, if these are indicated.

Concerns with opioids in the veterinary clinic

Opioids are the most effective drugs available for the control of acute pain in the dog and cat and yet many practices do not use them because they are concerned with the regulatory aspects or abuse potential of these drugs – most of the opioids are covered by some regulations, even though the agonist/antagonist drugs have very low abuse potential. However, as medical care professionals, it is incumbent on us to find solutions to this issue so that we can use the most effective therapies for our patients. Not wanting to do the 'paperwork' is an excuse that would be hard to explain to most clients. In many of these situations it is quite feasible to develop a solution which will ensure the safety of the drugs. One approach is for each veterinarian to have a locked container within another locked cupboard such that the practitioner is the only one with the key or combination. This ensures that no one else has access to those drugs. This would not prevent someone breaking into the practice to steal the drugs and if this is a problem for that locale it may be necessary to do without any controlled drugs. In some larger veterinary hospitals and in many human hospitals dispensing machines are used which will dispense specific doses of a drug when the correct access codes are entered. This can still not prevent abuse but it certainly reduces the chances since each entry is coded to the person entering it, therefore making it easier to identify any person who is abusing the system. As yet such machines are too expensive for individual practices. If opioids cannot be used then techniques combining local anaesthetics and NSAIDs should be developed.

Sensitivity to NSAIDs

Some animals have a sensitivity to NSAIDs – this may manifest as a gastrointestinal upset or the drugs may be relatively toxic to that individual (e.g. hepatic failure with carprofen, which has been reported in North America) (MacPhail et al 1998). Since the NSAIDs are the mainstay of chronic analgesic therapy this can make it very difficult to treat these patients. If the animal has shown a sensitivity to a particular drug then it may be possible to use a different NSAID without inducing the same side-effects. With the recent development of newer drugs which are more specific for COX-2, it may be expected that some of these side-effects will be reduced, but the full benefit of these drugs will not be understood until they have been in use for some time. For animals with cancer pain or other short-term non-arthritic pain, it may be feasible to use oral preparations of morphine (Dohoo et al 1994, Dohoo & Tasker 1997). Some of the slow release preparations can be used twice daily very effectively. Some dogs may not tolerate the morphine either (vomiting) but it is worth assessing to see if it will provide adequate pain relief.

Patients receiving monoamine oxidase inhibitors

Recently, selegiline, a non-competitive inhibitor of monoamine oxidase B, has been prescribed for ageing and for pituitary-dependent hyperadrenocorticism in dogs. This drug has been associated with severe reactions when human patients receiving chronic treatment have been given some opioids. The responses seen include hyperpyrexia, coma, severe hypertension, seizures and delirium (Zornberg et al 1991) and some of these cases have had a fatal outcome

173

(Mealey & Matthews 1999). The opioids most commonly associated with this reaction are pethidine/meperidine and pentazocine. Individual patients have been successfully given some of the more potent μ agonists (O'Hara et al 1995), e.g. fentanyl (Noorily et al 1997) but there have also been severe reactions associated with other monoamine oxidase inhibitors and fentanyl (Noble & Baker 1992, Insler et al 1994). Until more data become available on the likely interactions between selegiline and opioids, the clinician should avoid their combined use if possible. If opioids need to be used, then morphine and fentanyl appear to be the drugs of choice but the doses should be titrated carefully and discontinued if any untoward effects are seen. Pain management may be achieved more safely by the use of local anaesthetics and NSAIDs if these can be used appropriately.

Use of local anaesthetics

As discussed throughout this text, local anaesthetics can be used to provide preemptive and postoperative analgesia. In man it is common for local anaesthetics to be given with the patient awake because the anaesthesiologist is concerned about creating nerve damage with the technique. When a needle comes in contact with a nerve the patient experiences sensations coming from the area of innervation which can vary from tingling, to pain, to numbness. These sensations are referred to as paraesthesias and give the clinician a good indication that an injection at that site may cause damage to the nerve. Most of the local anaesthetic blocks used to control pain in dogs and cats are likely to be administered to the anaesthetised animal and so there is no such feedback (Pascoe 1997). Even when the animal is awake it is hard to determine the cause of a behavioural response to needle puncture and manipulation – is it just the normal sensation from the needle or is the animal reacting to a paraesthesia? Because of this lack of feedback it is important for the clinician to be very careful with the technique of injection and to ensure that the needle is placed accurately and carefully. Ideally a relatively 'blunt' needle should be used. Spinal needles have a much less sharp bevel than ordinary hypodermic needles and are preferred when doing major nerve blocks. It is also better to orient the bevel of the needle along the fibres of the nerve rather than across them. With this technique, if the nerve is penetrated, the neurones will tend to be separated rather than cut.

Local anaesthetics also block all sensation from the area which they are affecting. This means that the animal has no ability to know what has happened to that part of the body and damage may ensue. If a mandibular alveolar block is carried out and the lingual nerves are also blocked the tongue will be numb and the animal may cause serious damage to the tongue as it wakes up. If the animal has had a limb blocked it may put it in an awkward position and end up damaging the surgery site or even breaking a bone. Because of these issues it is important to monitor the patient carefully after the use of local anaesthetics so that self-inflicted injuries can be prevented.

References

Boatwight, C.E., Fubini, S.L.F., Groh, Y.T. et al (1996) A comparison of N-butylscopolammonium bromide and butorphanol tartrate for analgesia using a balloon model of abdominal pain in ponies. *Canadian Journal of Veterinary Research* **60**: 65–68.

Campbell, J.N. (1996) Complex regional pain syndrome and the sympathetic nervous system. In: Campbell, J.N. (ed) *Pain 1996 – An Updated Review*. International Association for the Study of Pain Press, Seattle, pp 89–96.

Cervero, F. (1999) Physiology and Physiopathology of Visceral Pain. In: Max, M. (ed) *Pain 1999 – An updated Review*. International Association for the Study of Pain Press, Seattle, pp 39–46.

Dellemijn, P. (1999) Are opioids effective in relieving neuropathic pain? *Pain* **80**: 453–462.

Dohoo, S.E. and Tasker, R.A. (1997) Pharmacokinetics of oral morphine sulfate in dogs: a comparison of sustained release and conventional formulations. *Canadian Journal of Veterinary Research* **61**: 251–255.

Dohoo, S., Tasker, R.A. and Donald, A. (1994) Pharmacokinetics of parenteral and oral sustained-release morphine sulphate in dogs. *Journal of Veterinary Pharmacology and Therapeutics* **17**: 426–433.

Field, M.J., McCleary, S., Hughes, J. et al (1999) Gabapentin and pregabalin, but not morphine and amitryptyline, block both static and dynamic components of mechanical allodynia induced by streptozocin in the rat. *Pain* **80**: 391–398.

Hay, W.P. and Moore, J.N. (1997) Management of pain in horses with colic. *Compendium on Continuing Education for the Practicing Veterinarian* **19**. 987–990.

Hinshaw, L.B., Beller, B.K., Chang, A.C.K. et al (1984) Evaluation of naloxone for therapy of *Escherichia coli* shock. *Archives of Surgery* **119**: 1410–1418.

Hunt, L.B., Gurll, N.J. and Reynolds, D.G. (1984) Dose-dependent effects of nalbuphine in canine hemorrhagic shock. *Circulation and Shock* **13**: 307–318.

Insler, S.R., Kraenzler, E.J., Licina, M.G. et al. (1994) Cardiac surgery in a patient taking monoamine oxidase inhibitors: an adverse fentanyl reaction. *Anesthesia and Analgesia* **78**: 593–597.

Irving, G.A. (1997) Acute pancreatitis. *Anesthesiology Clinics of North America* **15**: 319–334.

Isenhower, H. and Mueller, B. (1998) Selection of narcotic analgesics for pain associated with pancreatitis. *American Journal of Health-System Pharmacy* **55**: 480–486.

Jensen, T.S. (1996) Mechanisms of neuropathic pain. In: Campbell, J.N. (ed) *Pain 1996 – An Updated Review*. International Association for the Study of Pain Press, Seattle, pp 77–86.

Jochle, W. (1989) Field trial evaluation of detomidine as a sedative and analgesic in horses with colic. *Equine Veterinary Journal* (Suppl): 117–120.

Jochle, W., Moore, J., Brown, J. et al (1989) Comparison of detomidine, butorphanol, flunixin meglumine and xylazine in clinical cases of equine colic. *Equine Veterinary Journal* (Suppl): 111–116.

Joubert, K. (1998) Ketamine hydrochloride – an adjunct for analgesia in dogs with burn wounds. *Journal of the South African Veterinary Medical Association* **69**: 95–97.

Juvara, I. and Radulesco, D. (1967) Modifications of the contractility of the sphincter of Oddi under the influence of central analgesics (in French). *Revue Internationale D'Hepatologie* **17**: 55–63.

Kalpravidh, M., Lumb, W.V., Wright, M. et al (1984) Effects of butorphanol, morphine, and xylazine in ponies. *American Journal of Veterinary Research* **45**: 217–223.

Kohn, C.W. (1999) Medical Therapy for Gastrointestinal Diseases. In: Colahan, P.T., Mayhew, I.G., Merritt, A.M. et al (eds) *Equine Medicine and Surgery*, 5th edition. Mosby, St Louis, pp 603–638.

Kowalske, K.J. and Tanelian, D.T. (1997) Burn pain. *Anesthesiology Clinics of North America* **15**: 269–283.

Lascelles, B.D., Cripps, P., Mirchandani, S. et al (1995) Carprofen as an analgesic for postoperative pain in cats: dose titration and assessment of efficacy in comparison to pethidine hydrochloride. *Journal of Small Animal Practice* **36**: 535–541.

Lauretti, G.R., Lima, I.C.P.R., Resi, M.P. et al. (1999) Oral ketamine and transdermal nitroglycerin as analgesic adjuvants to oral morphine therapy for cancer pain management. *Anesthesiology* **90**: 1528–1533.

Lowe, J.E. (1978) Xylazine, pentazocine, meperidine, and dipyrone for relief of balloon induced equine colic: A double blind comparative evaluation. *Journal of Equine Medicine and Surgery* **2**: 286–291.

McCammon, R.L., Stoelting, R.K. and Madura, J.A. (1984) Effects of butorphanol, nalbuphine, and fentanyl on intrabiliary tract dynamics. *Anesthesia and Analgesia* **63**: 139–142.

McKellar, Q.A., Pearson, T., Bogan, J.A. et al (1990) Pharmacokinetics, tolerance and serum thromboxane inhibition of carprofen in the dog. *Journal of Small Animal Practice* **31**: 443–448.

MacPhail, C.M., Lappin, M.R., Meyer, D.J. et al (1998) Hepatocellular toxicosis associated with administration of carprofen in 21 dogs. *Journal of the American Veterinary Medical Association* **212**: 1895–1901.

Martin, S., Farr, L. and Murray, E. (1995) Clinical use of detomidine hydrochloride. *Equine Practice* **17**: 21–26, 29.

Mealey, K.A. and Matthews, N.S. (1999) Drug interactions during anesthesia. *Veterinary Clinics of North America: Small Animal Practice* **29**: 629–643.

Melzack, R., Wall, P.D. and Ty, T.C. (1982) Acute pain in an emergency clinic: latency of onset and descriptor patterns related to different injuries. *Pain* **14**: 33–43.

Merren, M.D. (1998) Gabapentin for treatment of pain and tremor: a large case series. *Southern Medical Journal* **91**: 739–744.

Noble, W.H. and Baker, A. (1992) MAO inhibitors and coronary artery surgery: a patient death. *Canadian Journal of Anaesthesia* **39**: 1061–1066.

Noorily, S., Hantler, C. and Sako, E. (1997) Monoamine oxidase inhibitors and cardiac anaesthesia revisited. *Southern Medical Journal* **90**: 836–838.

O'Hara, J., Maurer, W. and Smith, M. (1995) Sufentanil-isoflurane-nitrous oxide anesthesia for a patient treated with monoamine oxidase inhibitor and tricyclic antidepressant. *Journal of Clinical Anaesthesia* **7**: 148–150.

Pascoe, P.J. (1997) Local and regional anesthesia and analgesia. *Seminars in Veterinary Medicine and Surgery (Small Animal)* **12**: 94–105.

Robbins, W., Staats, P., Levine, J. et al (1998) Treatment of intractable pain with topical large-dose capsaicin: preliminary report. *Anesthesia and Analgesia* **86**: 579–583.

Roger, T., Bardon, T. and Ruckebusch, Y. (1994) Comparative effects of mu and kappa opiate antagonists on the cecocolic motility in the pony. *Canadian Journal of Veterinary Research* **58**: 163–166.

Rothuizen, J., de Vries-Chalmers Hoynck van Papendrecht, R. and van den Brom, W.E. (1990) Post prandial and cholecystokinin-induced emptying of the gall bladder in dogs. *Veterinary Record* **126**: 505–507.

Rowbotham, M., Harden, N., Stacey, B. et al (1998) Gabapentin for the treatment of postherpetic neuralgia: a randomized controlled trial. *Journal of the American Medical Association* **280**: 1837–1842.

Schafer, A.I. (1995) Effects of nonsteroidal antiinflammatory drugs on platelet function and systemic hemostasis. *Journal of Clinical Pharmacology* **35**: 209–219.

Stoneham, M.D., Cooper, R., Quiney, N.F. et al (1996) Pain following craniotomy: a preliminary study comparing PCA morphine with intramuscular codeine phosphate. *Anaesthesia* **51**: 1176–1178.

Takahashi, H., Miyazaki, M., Nanbu, T. et al (1998) NMDA-receptor antagonist ketamine abolishes neuropathic pain after epidural administration in a clinical case. *Pain* **75**: 391–394.

Taylor, P.M. and Clarke K.W. (1999) Handbook of Equine Anaesthesia. Bailliére Tindall, London.

Taylor, P.M., Delatour, P., Landoni, F.M. et al (1996) Pharmacodynamics and enantioselective pharmacokinetics of carprofen in the cat. *Research in Veterinary Science* **60**: 144–151.

van den Brock, A.H.M. (1991) Treatment of burns in dogs. *Veterinary Annual* **31**: 204–212.

Vatashsky, E., Beilin, B. and Aronson, H.B. (1984) Common bile duct pressure in dogs after opiate injection – epidural versus intravenous route. *Canadian Anaesthestists Society Journal* **31**: 650–653.

Waterman, A.E. and Kalthum, W. (1992) Use of opioids in providing postoperative analgesia in the dog: a double-blind trial of pethidine, pentazocine, buprenorphine, and butorphanol. In: Short, C.E. and Van Poznack, A. (eds) *Animal Pain*. Churchill Livingstone, New York, pp 466–479.

Yaksh, T.L. and Chaplan, S.R. (1997) Physiology and pharmacology of neuropathic pain. *Anesthesiology Clinics of North America* **15**: 335–352.

Zornberg, G., Bodkin, J. and Cohen, B. (1991) Severe adverse interaction between pethidine and selegiline. *Lancet* **337**: 246.

INDEX